T5-BQA-751

RJ 496 .S74 B57 1988
Bloom, Beth-Ann.
  A parent's guide to spina bifida

A Parent's
Guide to
SPINA
BIFIDA

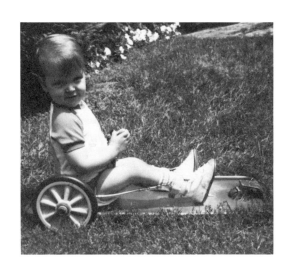

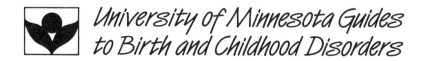 *University of Minnesota Guides to Birth and Childhood Disorders*

Edited by Robert J. Gorlin
Regents Professor of Oral Pathology and Genetics,
and Professor of Pediatrics, University of Minnesota

Advisory Board

David M. Brown, dean, Medical School, University of Minnesota

Judith G. Hall, Medical Genetics, University of British Columbia

Luanna H. Meyer, Special Education and Rehabilitation, Syracuse University

Margaret O'Dougherty, Neurology, Children's Hospital, Columbus, Ohio

Paul Quie, Pediatrics, University of Minnesota

Maynard Reynolds, Special Education Program, Education Psychology, University of Minnesota

Muriel B. Ryden, School of Nursing, University of Minnesota

Joe Leigh Simpson, Clinical Genetics, Obstetrics and Gynecology, University of Tennessee, Memphis

Joseph Warshaw, Pediatrics, Yale Medical School, New Haven

Subjects of Forthcoming Volumes

Cerebral palsy	Heart disorders	Sickle-cell anemia
Cleft lip and palate	Kidney disorders	and thalassemia
Cystic fibrosis	Leukemia	Spine deformities

A Parent's Guide to SPINA BIFIDA

Beth-Ann Bloom, M.S., Genetic Counselor, Gillette Childrens' Hospital, St. Paul, MN

Edward L. Seljeskog, M.D., Professor of Neurosurgery, University of Minnesota Medical School, Minneapolis, MN

University of Minnesota Press, Minneapolis

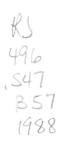

Copyright © 1988 by the University of Minnesota. All rights reserved.
No part of this publication may be reproduced, stored in a retrieval
system, or transmitted, in any form or by any means, electronic,
mechanical, photocopying, recording, or otherwise, without the prior
written permission of the publisher.

Published by the University of Minnesota Press, 2037 University Avenue
Southeast, Minneapolis, MN 55414. Published simultaneously in Canada
by Fitzhenry & Whiteside Limited, Markham. Printed in the United
States of America.

Library of Congress Cataloging-in-Publication Data

Bloom, Beth-Ann.
  A parent's guide to spina bifida.
  (University of Minnesota guides to birth and childhood disorders)
    Bibliography: p.
    Includes index.
    1. Spina bifida—Popular works. 2. Spina bifida—Complications
and sequelae. I. Seljeskog, Edward L.
II. Title. III. Series.
RJ496.S74B57 1988 618.92'8 88-10784
ISBN 0-8166-1486-5

The University of Minnesota
is an equal-opportunity
educator and employer.

CONTENTS

FOREWORD

A Parent's Guide to Spina Bifida is a volume in a series addressing the needs not only of parents but also of physicians and persons concerned with the care of children with relatively common disorders. We used as a model *The Child with Down's Syndrome*, written by David W. Smith, M.D., and Ann Asper Wilson and first published in 1973 by W. B. Saunders, Philadelphia. The book is very valuable because it makes the complex concepts of genetics and pediatrics understandable to parents. Such is the goal of our series.

In *A Parent's Guide to Spina Bifida* our authors discuss the various forms of failure of neural tube closure ranging from the always lethal anencephaly to the entirely benign spina bifida occulta. Attention is principally directed to the many aspects of spina bifida: causative factors, usual signs and symptoms, methods of diagnosis, early care, and the team approach to treatment. The authors address the questions most often asked: Why did it happen? Is it something for which we parents were at fault? What are the chances that it will happen if we have another child? What can we do to avoid its happening again? What can we expect in the way of complications? What can we do to help our child?

They have discussed in a lucid manner the possible problems faced by the affected child: hydrocephalus, lack of com-

plete bowel and bladder control, orthopedic concerns ranging from walking and the use of braces to hip dislocation and
spinal curvature. In the final section, such sensitive issues as
special educational facilities and problems of growing up are
addressed: self-image, independence, and sexuality and its
possible outcome, pregnancy. The authors have added a
very useful appendix to help the reader understand technical
terms, become acquainted with community and national
resources, and know of other books which may answer additional questions.

This book was written by Beth-Ann Bloom, M.S., and
Edward L. Seljeskog, M.D., Ph.D. Beth-Ann Bloom is pres-
ently genetic counselor for Gillette Children's Hospital and
St. Paul Ramsey Medical Center, St. Paul, Minnesota. She
received an M.S. degree in human genetics from Sarah Lawrence College, is a diplomate of the American Board of Medical Genetics, and is known for her teaching ability and sen-
sitivity to parents' problems.

Dr. Seljeskog is currently professor and vice chairman of
the Department of Neurosurgery, School of Medicine, University of Minnesota. He received his graduate training in
general surgery and neurological surgery at the University of
Minnesota and the University of Oslo. Dr. Seljeskog has
served on a large number of national and international neurosurgical committees and has several dozen publications to
his credit.

The need for this series is obvious. Parents of a child with
a serious disability need answers. They need to know not
only the nature of their child's disorder but also its possible
causes, its prognosis, the limitations it will impose on the
child, the impact it will have on the entire family, and the
chances of its recurring in either the parents' future children
or in the affected child's children. And, certainly, they need
to know what they themselves can do to help.

In spite of good intentions, the health professional has not
always been an effective communicator. These books are
designed to open the lines of communication between the
health professional and parents by increasing parents' un-

derstanding and providing them with a basic vocabulary for easier and more accurate expression of the worries, doubts, and uncertainties attendant on each disorder. It is our intention that health professionals play a vital part by supplementing each text with their own expertise. We cannot hope to answer all the questions that may be posed by parents, but we believe that each book will go a long way toward answering many of the common ones.

R. J. G.

INTRODUCTION

"I'm sorry, but your baby has spina bifida" are very confusing words to parents who were anticipating the birth of a healthy baby. Many people have never heard of spina bifida and the other neural tube defects. Most people know very little about them.

Our purpose in writing this book was to explain more about spina bifida and the other neural tube defects, to assist parents and relatives in absorbing the wealth of medical information and facts available about spina bifida and the conditions associated with it. We chose to make the style informal, attempting to keep to a minimum medical terminology and complex technical explanations. However, we do use some of the medical vocabulary applied to spina bifida and have provided a glossary at the back of the book where we define these words. It was our hope that by presenting simple, practical explanations of a very complex medical condition we would enable parents to more knowledgeably participate in medical decision-making about their child. The most essential element in successfully treating this demanding medical problem and effectively dealing with its many social and vocational implications is that parents play a key role in fostering the best in medical and supportive care for their child.

As you read this book, we would like you to keep in mind that just as every newborn is unique, is different from everyone else, so too every child with a birth defect is a unique individual. All children with the same diagnosis do not have every feature in common. Because all children are different, their medical treatment will vary. It is important to cherish the individuality of each child and to remember that no single statement applies to every child who has the same medical condition.

A Parent's Guide to
SPINA
BIFIDA

Chapter 1
WHAT IS SPINA BIFIDA?

Think of the very complex structure of the brain as the most powerful computer we know. It is built from genetic or hereditary blueprints that are invisible even under most ordinary microscopes. Its framework is assembled quickly over a few days and then developed, modified, and expanded over the following weeks. If even one small piece is altered or damaged in transit, there is no chance to go back to the stockroom to find a replacement. The brain controls all parts of the intricate physical structure we know as the human body. Its major line of communication with the body is the spinal cord, the cord of nerve tissue extending through the spinal column. When you think of the brain as a very complicated computer and the spinal cord as its primary connection or cable to the rest of the body, it's easy to imagine how something can so easily go wrong in its creation and development, and how a minor change or alteration in the nerves of the spinal cord can cause so many problems for a child.

Most of the information in this book is about children with spina bifida. Spina bifida is the most easily spelled and pronounced name for a group of serious birth defects of the central nervous system, which is composed of the brain and spinal cord. Spina bifida is often referred to as a *neural tube defect* or NTD.

What Is Spina Bifida?

There are several kinds of spina bifida. One is known as **spina bifida cystica,** a general term for a group of conditions that are referred to as **myelomeningocele**, **meningomyelocele**, and **myelodysplasia**. All of these terms refer to a birth defect in which a portion of the spinal cord and its nearby nerves have failed to develop normally. Instead of remaining inside the back, within the bony protection of the vertebrae of the spine, a portion of the spinal cord and some of the nerves are on the surface of the baby's back, usually in the lower (lumbar) spinal area, toward the middle or midline area. Most often the area of the maldeveloped spinal cord and nerves is enclosed in a thin-walled sac or cyst containing spinal fluid, hence the medical term "cystica." Most of the nerves originating from or going to this abnormal spinal cord area are impaired. As a consequence, these nerves often do not function normally.

In another type of spina bifida cystica, there is only an abnormality of the bony spinal canal, with a fluid-filled sac protruding from the surface of the skin. The spinal cord and nerves are not involved, maldeveloped, or damaged. As a consequence, the legs and bladder function normally. This lesser type of congenital spinal defect is called a *meningocele*.

Finally, there is another common abnormality, **spina bifida occulta**, which should not be confused with the two kinds of spina bifida cystica. Spina bifida occulta refers to a minor, purely bony abnormality involving only a defect or gap in a portion of one of the covering bones **(lamina)** of the vertebrae of the spine. There is no sac nor is there any nerve or spinal-cord involvement. It is a fairly common minor abnormality and is found in perhaps 5% of the population. It is most often noted only on an x-ray of the spine. Because the nerves and spinal cord are completely normal, spina bifida occulta is not truly a neural tube defect and may not be genetically linked to these defects. Individuals with spina bifida occulta do not have the medical problems we will be discussing in this book.

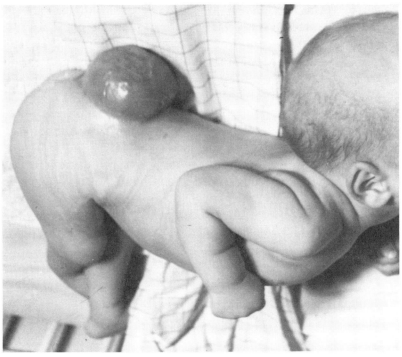

FIGURE 1.
A typical lumbo-sacral myelomeningocele sac in the lower back area. The baby's hips are flexed, making it impossible for him to straighten or extend his legs.

We will use the terms spina bifida, myelodysplasia, meningomyelocele, and myelomeningocele interchangeably. Often different terms are used in different regions of the country. You should feel free to choose whichever term you choose to, but become comfortable with all of them.

Perhaps the best place to begin is with a picture of a myelomeningocele (Figure 1) taken several days after the baby was born. In the middle of the infant's lower back is the thin myelomeningocele sac filled with spinal fluid. On the surface of the sac and within it are the maldeveloped end of the spinal cord and the damaged nerves. Most myelomeningoceles are quite obvious in the delivery room at the time of birth. Most often, the pregnancy has gone quite normally, so the parents and the health professionals are usually very surprised. Many parents will remember a hush falling over the delivery room, as the nurses and doctor noted the abnormality and examined the baby.

The newborn is usually taken immediately to the nursery, sometimes even before the parents see the baby or know if it's a boy or girl. If the baby is born in a small general hospital, arrangements are frequently made for the baby to be transferred to a larger facility with a Newborn Intensive Care Unit (NICU), where neurosurgical consultants are available. These types of special nurseries are designed to care for babies who have birth defects, who are very sick, or who are born prematurely. Many times a transport team of doctors or nurses will be called to pick the baby up to bring it safely to the Newborn Intensive Care Unit, which may be some miles distant. They will also stay in touch with the family and help make arrangements for the parents to come to be with the baby.

Every family reacts differently to the news that their baby has a birth defect. There is no right or wrong way. Often parents are so shocked they feel numb. Or they may cry—tears are common. Many parents feel angry. And they often ask, "Why me?" Some parents want nothing to do with the baby, while others refuse to leave their newborn's side. During this time, parents need much support from their own families, their friends, and the health-care team.

What Kind of Treatment Is Available?

When the baby arrives in the Newborn Intensive Care Unit, everything is checked to be certain that the baby is not in distress and is in stable condition—breathing regularly, with a normal blood pressure and pulse, warm enough, etc. The baby is examined by a pediatrician or perhaps a neonatologist—a pediatrician with a special interest in the care of the newborn. He or she will also look for any other medical problems. Many pediatric intensive-care units are in teaching hospitals where there are also interns, residents, and medical students, all of whom are part of the team taking care of the baby. Since spina bifida is relatively rare, they all may not be that familiar with the condition, but they will be working with more experienced doctors and other specialists to get information. These members of the team will have a major role in the baby's day-to-day general care. Finally, and most important, are the nurses in the special nurseries who are experts in answering parents' questions. They are professionals who can help families feel comfortable at a very stressful time. All members of this pediatric team expect to be asked questions, so parents should not be reluctant to speak out. With this unusual and complicated medical condition, there are no foolish questions. And there are many questions without precise or clearcut answers.

During this initial period, the baby will have many tests and examinations to determine the extent of the damage to the exposed spinal cord and the nerves, and to look for additional complications or other birth defects. Usually the baby will be kept lying on its stomach or side, to prevent pressure on the thin-walled sac. Often the baby will be kept in an isolette, a small, plastic-enclosed baby bed, in an attempt to provide the infant with extra warmth and protection. If the sac is thin-walled, it is often kept covered with something moist and sterile, since any opening into the sac puts the baby at risk for a very serious infection of the spinal fluid (**meningitis**).

In addition to the pediatrician and other specialists, a neurosurgical consultant or neurosurgeon is involved in these early examinations. Neurosurgeons are specialists on surgery of the brain and spinal cord. Some neurosurgeons are so highly specialized that they work only with children—pediatric neurosurgeons. A neurologist or pediatric neurologist may also be part of the team. These specialists are ex-

perts on the nonsurgical and developmental problems of the
nervous system.

Among the tests the baby will have shortly after being ad-
mitted to the nursery is an x-ray of the spine, which will
show which vertebrae are involved in the defect. Additional
tests will also be done to see if the baby has **hydrocephalus**.
This is a serious problem that develops in many children
with spina bifida. The tests for this condition include: ultrasound or **CT (Computerized Tomography)** scans of the
baby's head, which often reveal the presence and degree of
severity of the hydrocephalus.

At this initial examination, there is usually some evidence
of weakness in the baby's ankles or legs, owing to the damaged nerves in the myelomeningocele sac. Often it is hard to
see more than a bit of weakness at the foot or ankle, but on
occasion, when the abnormality is large, both legs can be
completely paralyzed.

At birth, many infants with myelodysplasia have obvious
deformities of their feet or legs. This happens because the
nerve damage prevents the baby's legs from moving normally within the uterus. Some muscles contract normally,
while others are weak or paralyzed. Although these deformities may cause problems as time goes on, they often cannot
be completely evaluated and treated until the baby is old
enough to cooperate with the examination. Another area
that gets only a quick initial look is the newborn's bowel and
bladder control. It will be important to know that the baby
urinates and passes stool, but other more formal testing
won't be done until a bit later.

The most important immediate decision in the first day of
life is what to do about the thin-walled sac or large open area
on the baby's back. Many years ago, there was nothing that
could be done. Most of these babies eventually died from
overwhelming infection. Now this can usually be prevented.

After evaluating the baby's physical condition, nerve function, and the degree of hydrocephalus, if any, the neurosurgeon and other members of the health-care team will contact
the parents. They will give their best estimate of which of

any related problems the baby will have in the future. Although they will be using their best judgment and the best information available, it is still often difficult to precisely answer many of the questions about the infant's future.

After presenting their information and conclusions to the parents, the doctors and others involved will usually recommend that the baby have surgery, often immediately, for repair and closing of the myelomeningocele sac and will ask for the parents' consent to this operation. The members of the team know that this is a very difficult time for the family. They try to respond to all of the family's questions and concerns so that the parents will be comfortable in giving their permission for the operation. On rare occasions, when the defect is large and severe or when other abnormalities are present, the medical professionals will state that the baby's future is so hopeless that only supportive general care should be given and that an operation would not be wise or appropriate. Parents should always freely ask questions at this time and have a full and complete understanding of the reasons for any of the recommendations. Most important, they should fully agree with the doctors' advice. If the recommendation is for supportive care only (no surgery), the parents should understand why this recommendation is being made and be in complete agreement with it. If they are not, they should feel free to ask for additional evaluation or even a second opinion. After hearing the outlook for their baby's future, occasionally parents feel the required care and the child's handicap will be more than they can handle. They may wish to learn more about the option of placing the baby for foster care or adoption. There are a number of individuals and families who are very willing to care for or adopt babies with spina bifida.

During the initial operation, the neurosurgeon repairs and closes the baby's back. The nerves are tucked back inside the spinal canal, and layer by layer the tissues and the skin are carefully closed over them. This operation accomplishes several things: it removes and closes the sac, stops any leakage of spinal fluid, reduces the chance of infection, and prevents further nerve damage. It is important to remember that the damage already done to the spinal cord cannot be corrected, even with modern techniques.

Most often this initial surgery is done in the first day or so of the baby's life. Frequently it is done on a semi-emergency basis. Occasionally, when the sac already has a complete thick covering of normal skin, the operation can be safely delayed. The surgery is usually routine and lasts about one to two hours.

After the operation, the infant returns to the special-care nursery. As the baby's back begins to heal, the parents will finally get a chance to hold their child. During this time, the baby's condition will be closely monitored to check for problems, especially for infection around the surgical area and for the development of hydrocephalus. When everything is healed and stable, and there are no other concerns, the infant can leave the hospital. This period of time varies in length depending upon whether there are any complications following surgery or whether other problems develop. On average it is about 10 days.

What Will Be the Result of Damaged Nerves?

Much of the testing of the baby in the nursery is done to determine how much nerve damage there is. The predictions about his or her future hinge on the extent of the damage. Before discussing what this means for a child with spina bifida, let's review how nerves work.

There are many misconceptions about nerves. Such common expressions as "You really get on my nerves" and "I have a lot of nervous energy" imply that nerves are involved with emotions and a person's degree of energy. This isn't an accurate medical definition of nerves or how they function.

Nerves are the major way in which the brain communicates with the rest of the body. Essentially, the nerves create a two-way communications network, almost like a telephone system. If the brain wants something done, it uses the nerves to relay a message to a muscle or group of muscles. For example, if you want to put your finger on your nose, you can precisely send a message along the nerves to your shoulder, arm, hand, and finger to move onto your nose. Once your finger gets there, other nerves can send back messages to say that "this feels like a nose." At the same time, the nerves on your nose can transmit messages to your brain that say "we sense there is a finger on us." While all this is going on, remember that other nerves are simultaneously making your eyes see the people who are pointing at the foolish person poised with finger on nose and your ears hear their laughter (Figure 2). The brain is indeed a complex computer.

There are two basic types of nerves. Motor nerves arise from the spinal cord and relay messages from the brain via the spinal cord, telling the muscles to move the bones and joints. Sensory nerves send messages back to the spinal cord and then to the brain, telling the brain what the other parts of the body are sensing or feeling. Typically, the motor nerve pathways travel from the brain to its base and downward into the spinal cord. From there they connect at each level of the spine to other parts of the body, via nerves. Each emerging motor nerve is responsible for movement of a particular muscle or a particular part of the body. Each spinal level also has a set of entering sensory nerves, from a particular body area or region of skin surface. These sensory pathways enter the spinal cord where they ascend to the skull base and from there to the brain.

An easy way to think about this is to say that the nerves from the neck (cervical) area of the spinal cord go to the upper part of the body and to the arms; those from the center (thoracic) region go to the trunk and abdomen; and nerves from the bottom or tail end of the spinal cord (lumbar and sacral) go to the lower part of the body, including the legs, bladder, and rectum. Specific medical terminology is used to explain which nerves go where. It is fairly technical, but

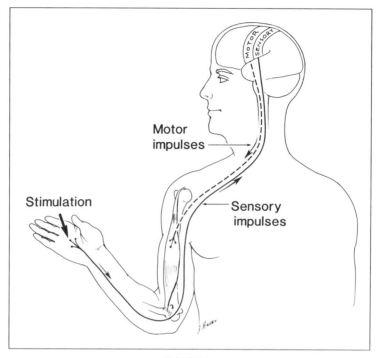

FIGURE 2.
A typical motor nerve pathway conducting nerve impulses from the brain to an arm muscle. Also, a typical sensory nerve pathway conducting pain or touch sensation from the hand to the spinal cord and the brain.

since it is widely used when talking about spina bifida, it is worth knowing a bit about. Nerves are given the names of the vertebrae they pass when leaving the spinal cord. At the top of the spine are the seven cervical vertebrae, numbered from the top down as Cervical 1 through 7 (C1-C7); next come the twelve thoracic or chest area vertebrae labeled Thoracic 1 through 12 (T1-T12); and finally are the five lumbar (L1-L5) and five sacral elements (S1-S5). The diagram (Figure 3) shows the areas supplied by particular nerves. With this introduction to nerves you can now perhaps better under-

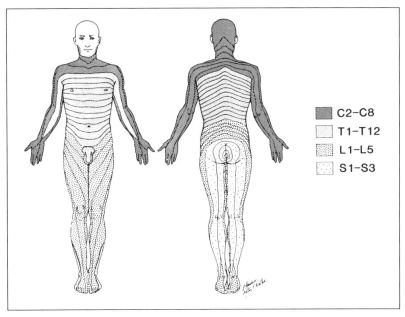

FIGURE 3.
The usual pattern of spinal-nerve distribution (dermatomes) to each body area. Note the areas stimulated by the cervical, thoracic, lumbar, and sacral nerves.

stand the neurological or nerve examination of the infant with myelodysplasia.

To examine the nerves of an adult, the physician asks the patient to perform certain motions, tell if a pinprick is felt, and cooperate with reflex testing. Babies cannot cooperate with any of these tests, so it is much more difficult to accurately examine their nerves. Instead of asking a baby to kick or raise a foot, the doctor must wait to see if the baby does it independently. Then the strength of the muscles can be evaluated. The sensory nerves are often checked by pricking with a pin or a small pinch to see if the baby flinches. Bladder and bowel function are also influenced by sensory and motor nerves, so these areas are also checked during a neurological examination.

The point of all these tests on a baby with myelodysplasia is to find the spinal-cord level above which all of the nerves work and react normally and below which none of the nerves works. It is a search for the place where the telephone lines to and from the brain are damaged, so that messages cannot be sent any further up or down the spinal cord. This kind of examination was originally done on people who had suffered injuries which damaged their spinal cord during an accident. In most of these accident cases, it is fairly clear exactly which nerves are still working. The situation is often somewhat less distinct with children who have a meningomyelocele. Their spinal cord and nerves often do not have a precise demarcation between normal and abnormal, at least one that can be determined by the neurological exam, so that they may have more damage to the right side of the spinal cord than to the left (or vice versa) or there can be more motor loss than sensory loss (or the other way around too). For example, an examination may put a child's motor neurological level at L4, but there may still be some feeling in the feet, even though the diagram in Figure 3 may not lead you to predict this finding. After the neurological testing is done, parents may expect the doctors to predict things such as the child's ability to walk. At this stage, predictions like these cannot be done with great certainty or confidence. A baby may have nerves to encourage a muscle to move while he or she is lying down, but there may not be a powerful enough message to the muscle to permit the strength required for walking.

Even though there are many vertebrae, open spine defects seem to cluster in the lower (lumbar) area of the back. In a survey of 300 patients in Australia, 92% of the defects occurred below L2 and the largest percentage were found where the lumbar and sacral areas come together (L5 or S1). This finding is in keeping with the experience of other treatment centers.

In our introduction we said that each child with a neural tube defect is an individual. The wide range of functions, dependent on the level of nerve damage, is just one illustration of this uniqueness. Later we will discuss the significance of nerve damage as the child grows older.

How Did This Happen?

When a baby is born with a birth defect like spina bifida, many parents ask, "How did this happen, whose fault is it, and will it happen again?" These are very appropriate questions. The medical professionals best prepared to provide answers to these questions are medical geneticists and genetic counselors.

We don't fully understand the cause of neural tube defects, but it's not because we haven't tried to do so. There are several reasons why this has proved to be a difficult research problem.

The Role of Genes

The error that results in spina bifida occurs very early in pregnancy, before most women even realize they have conceived. By four weeks of gestation, the problem has to a large extent already happened. At this point in pregnancy the embryo looks more like a salamander than the baby it will become. All nerve tissue in the human embryo begins as a flat disc. The flattened disc area that will become the brain and spinal cord needs to form a groove that folds together to form a tube. This tube then needs to zip its edges together like a winter jacket. When this closure is not complete, a neural tube defect results. Many embryos with improperly closed neural tubes are too impaired or weakened to survive pregnancy and are miscarried. Miscarriages are more common in families where a child is born with myelomeningocele. However, this does not mean that every miscarriage in these families is of a fetus with a neural tube defect.

Because this folding error occurs so early in pregnancy, it makes the problem very difficult to study.

We know neural tube defects are caused partly by genetic factors. Most parents find this fact difficult to accept, since it hasn't happened previously in their family. Actually, 95% of babies with spina bifida are born into families where it has never occurred before.

An easy way to understand the genetic part of this problem is to remember that genes are the chemicals that give cells directions on the proper way to develop and grow. Genes give the embryo directions and guidance for proper folding and formation of the neural tube. Since the nervous system is so complex, several different genes work together to design and regulate its development.

Half of all a baby's genes come from its mother and half from its father. This is also true of the genes that form the neural tube. Although many relatives may say, "That came from their side, not ours," this is not usually true. Both parents contribute equally, so there is no point in blaming your spouse or feeling guilty yourself.

Because neural tube defects are partly genetic, they occur more frequently in families and in certain ethnic groups than would be expected if they were a random problem. While 1 to 2 of every 1,000 babies born in the United States have a neural tube defect, the problem is more common in Northern Ireland and Wales, where 8 of every 1,000 babies have a neural tube defect. When people emigrate from those countries to the United States, they bring their genes with them and also their chance of having a baby with a neural tube defect. The risk, however, drops to about 3 in 1,000. That gives us another way to understand how much of this birth defect is caused by genetic factors. This does not mean that if a parent has Irish or Welsh ancestors, it is his or her fault that the baby has spina bifida.

The fact that the emigrants who bring their genes along can ultimately change the original birth rates for myelomeningocele is evidence that neural tube defects are not solely genetic. They are also caused by other factors, including environmental ones. The precise nature of these factors is hard to identify. Since they affect a woman approximately nine months before the baby is born, it's hard to remember what she was exposed to so long before. Whatever these factors are, they must be fairly common since babies are born with neural tube defects all over the world.

Many theories have been proposed regarding which environmental factors are responsible. They are believed for a while and then proven wrong. This situation is frustrating for parents and for scientists trying to understand the problem. Some of the earlier theories were based on the observation that the problem was more common in Ireland. Potatoes, potato blight, and Irish whiskey were blamed. These theories were shown to be false. Also considered and abandoned for the most part were theories that blamed elevated maternal temperatures caused by infections or hot tubs.

The latest theory to be proposed suggests that a vitamin deficiency may lead to the problem. This theory is still being tested. Women should not take vitamins to prevent neural tube defects without medical advice, since excess vitamins can cause other fetal abnormalities.

Even though neither the genetic nor the environmental components of neural tube defects are fully understood, genetic counselors can provide useful information to most families. Geneticists will ask questions so they can draw a family tree. They will also check to see that the baby has the common type of spina bifida we have been reviewing and not one of the rarer forms associated with other birth defects. When this information is available, the genetic counselor can tell the family what chance there is that their next baby will have spina bifida. In all cases the best chance is that their next baby will be fine. For most couples the chance that it will happen again is around 3% to 5%. Since there are differences among families, it is important that families get individualized genetic counseling to learn more about their own risks.

Other family members may also want to know what their chances are for having a baby with spina bifida. They too can consult a genetic counselor. In general, the risks to the children of the aunts, uncles, brothers, and sisters of a baby with a neural tube defect are less than to the parents, but greater than to the general population.

In the past, genetic counselors could only advise parents of the estimates of recurrence risks. Now they can offer additional testing. These more specific tests during pregnancy will give further information about whether or not the fetus has a neural tube defect. Since most babies are healthy, these prenatal tests usually give reassuring news, and for this reason many parents choose to have the tests. Other couples decide against having them done. These are very personal decisions and should be made only when parents have complete information from their health-care providers.

One prenatal test for neural tube defects is based on an observation made by British researchers during the 1970s. They noted a substance in fetal blood called Alpha Feto Protein (AFP), a substance not found in adult blood. Normally a small amount of AFP passes from the fetus into the amniotic fluid or bag of waters surrounding it. When there is unprotected and uncovered spinal cord tissue, as in a neural tube defect, a lot more AFP than usual is found in the amniotic fluid.

Amniotic fluid can be safely removed from the mother's uterus by an experienced obstetrician trained in this technique. The procedure used to remove the fluid is called amniocentesis. AFP is usually best studied when the test is done some 15-17 weeks after the mother's last menstrual period. An ultrasound examination is done first. Sophisticated electronic equipment is used to produce high-frequency nonaudible sound waves which make a picture of the fetus. Structures in the fetal body can be identified and measured, and the safest place from which to take the amniotic fluid determined. The obstetrician then inserts a thin needle through the woman's abdominal wall and into her uterus so that a small amount of amniotic fluid can be withdrawn.

The AFP test results return from the lab in a few days. A normal result from an experienced laboratory is very reassuring that an open neural tube is probably not present. In the rare situation where the neural tube defect happens to be covered with skin, AFP testing cannot reveal the presence of the defect. If, however, the AFP level is high, other confirmatory tests can be done, and the parents will then be given as much information as is available about the fetus's condition as well as their future options.

Amniocentesis for AFP measurement should be offered to all parents who have had a child with a neural tube defect. Since spina bifida is normally not common in the general population, it is not a practical test to offer to all pregnant women. Furthermore, there are some small but definite risks to amniocentesis, which can be fully explained at the time of genetic counseling. There is now an additional test designed to determine which women have a higher chance of carrying a fetus with a neural tube defect and who should be offered amniocentesis. This test is called Maternal Serum AFP screening (MS-AFP). This screening takes advantage of the fact that small amounts of the AFP in the amniotic fluid do leak into the mother's bloodstream. We know the normal amount expected to be found for different weeks of gestation. Since this is a screening test, it is not as reliable for diagnosing a neural tube defect as is amniocentesis. But if there is a normal amount of AFP, the result is reassuring. An elevated serum value may require additional testing. For example, an ultrasound examination can provide further information. Perhaps the woman is carrying twins and two fetuses producing AFP are responsible for the elevation. At other times, the ultrasound shows the gestational age to be different from what was expected. If no easy answer is gained from the additional tests, the woman can be offered amniocentesis. In most cases, even with an elevated serum AFP in the mother's blood, the greatest chance is that the fetus is developing normally. It is important to get the best information possible when considering AFP testing.

What Other Neural Tube Defects Are There?

The most common neural tube defect to affect families is spina bifida, which is why most of this book has been devoted to myelomeningocele. However, we would like to briefly discuss two other neural tube defects, **anencephaly** and **encephalocele**.

Anencephaly

This is the abnormality that results when the neural tube fails to close at the top or head end rather than lower down the spine. Because the neural tube in the head region fails to close, the baby's brain does not form normally. It is a tragic defect. Infants with anencephaly cannot survive.

The pregnancy is often abnormal when a woman is carrying a fetus with anencephaly. Frequently there is an excessive amount of amniotic fluid, delivery is overdue, and labor can be prolonged. Many ancephalic babies are stillborn, though some may be born alive and continue to breathe for a short while. Since there is no brain, the skull does not form normally. Often the physician will suspect the pregnancy is abnormal and will request some tests. An ultrasound may show that the fetus is anencephalic. There is no treatment for this condition.

Hearing that a fetus is anencephalic is often devastating. Although the disorder occurs once in every 1,000 births, most people have never heard of it. The causes and the chance of it happening again are about the same as noted previously for spina bifida. At delivery parents may be given the opportunity to see and hold their newborn. Even though it may be very painful emotionally, this chance to see and perhaps say good-bye to their baby is the beginning of the healing process after this sad event.

Encephalocele

Encephalocele is another neural tube defect involving the brain. In this condition, although the skull closes, a sac protrudes from it, filled with spinal fluid. The sac may contain abnormally developed brain tissue. In North America and Europe, it is usually at the back of the skull. The amount of damage to the child varies; it relates to the amount of brain within the sac. Occasionally birth defects such as kidney malformations, extra fingers, or cleft palate are associated with this neural tube defect. Some of these children develop hydrocephalus. Given all these possibilities, the future of a child with an encephalocele is very difficult to predict. The chance of this problem happening again varies greatly. It can be as high as 25%. For this reason, parents of a child with an encephalocele are well-advised to see a genetic counselor.

Nicole is 8 months old and loves to play with her toys.

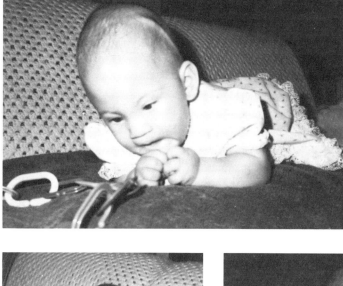

She has spina bifida, but does most things other babies her age do.

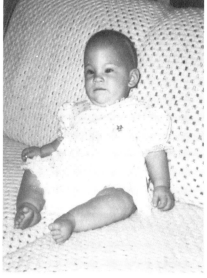

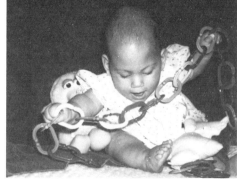

Nicole spent several weeks in the hospital when she was a newborn and has been back in to have her shunt replaced.

Nicole now has very little hair so you can see her shunt. When her hair grows in, the bump will be well hidden.

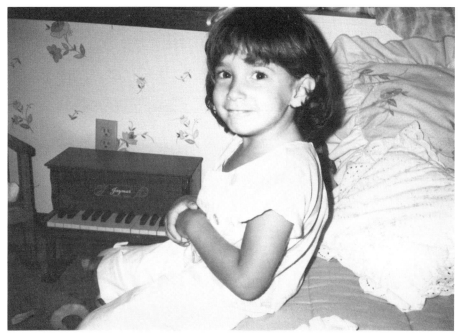

Like many 4-year-old girls, Jackie loves showing off her bedroom with its frilly pillows, toy piano, and dolls.

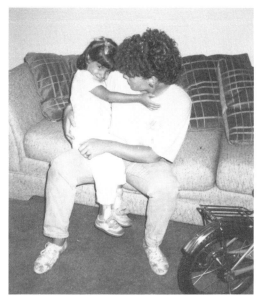

Cuddling with mommy and riding a two-wheeler are important to Jackie. Her mother started a support group in which mothers of children with spina bifida can talk to each other.

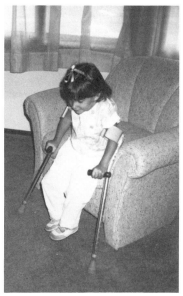

Her crutches help Jackie get around. Her myelomeningo-cele was at L-5.

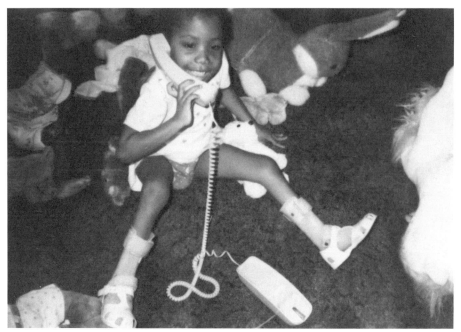

At 6 years old, bubbly Mechelle uses the phone and her AFOs (braces) to keep up with her friends.

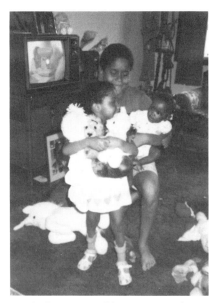

Mechelle is a good big sister and shares her toys.

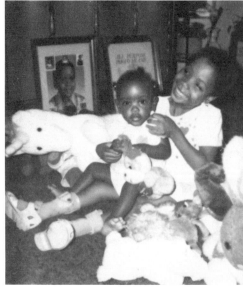

She may need extra help to keep up at school but Mechelle has no problem keeping up with her family.

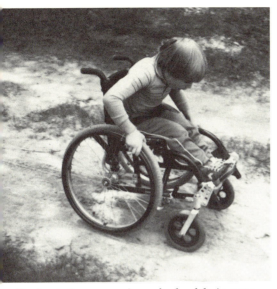

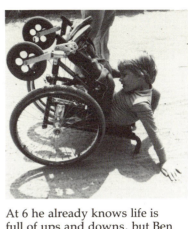

At 6 he already knows life is full of ups and downs, but Ben knows how to get his chair upright.

Benjamin is an experienced wheelchair racer who competes with both able-bodied and disabled adults and children.

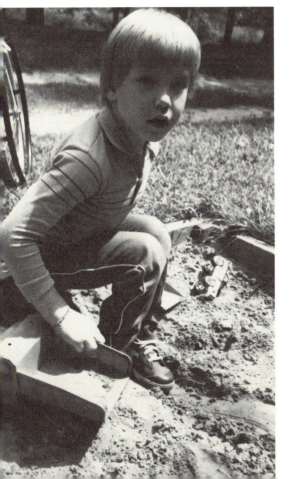

Kids with spina bifida can be as silly as any kids.

It's fun to climb out of your wheelchair and dig in the sand.

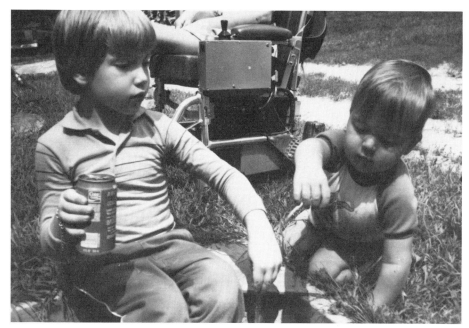

Ben's brother Nicholas is 2 years old.

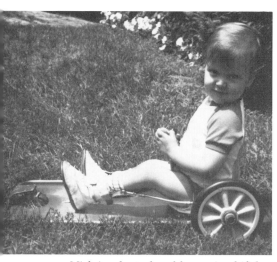

Nick is adopted and has spina bifida.

He tries very hard to follow in his big
brother's tracks.

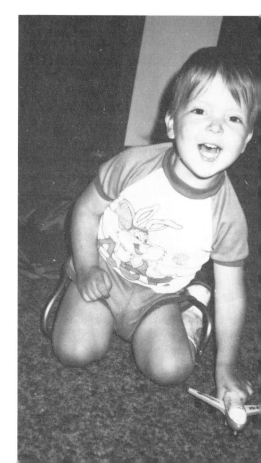

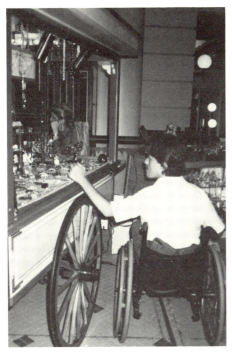

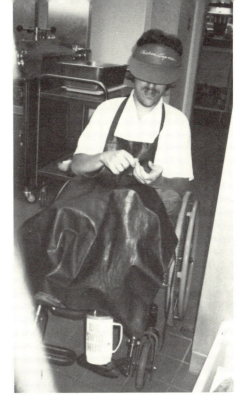

Jim is 24 years old and lives in his own apartment. Here he stops to do a little shopping on his way to work.

He works in a fast-food restaurant. Even while at work Jim keeps a cup of water handy, knowing the importance of drinking plenty of water daily.

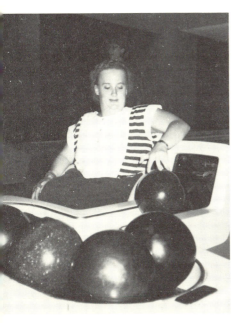

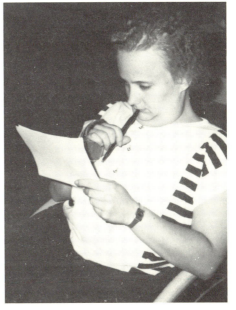

Cheryl is an avid (and very good) bowler on a team with able-bodied players.

This 25-year-old devotes considerable attention to her score sheet and to her office job.

Chapter 2
MEDICAL PROBLEMS ASSOCIATED WITH SPINA BIFIDA

Hydrocephalus

One problem that frequently develops in children with mye-lodysplasia is hydrocephalus. To understand this condition and its treatment it is helpful to know about the construction or anatomy of the brain. The roots of the word tell us that hydrocephalus involves a problem with water (hydro) and the brain (cephalus). In all individuals it is normal to have water, or more precisely spinal fluid (**cerebrospinal fluid** or CSF), within the brain cavities and in and around its surface. CSF protects the brain inside the skull the way the amniotic fluid protects the baby in the uterus, or the way the juice in a peach jar protects the peaches. Besides guarding the brain from drying out, and cushioning it against bruising, the CSF carries away wastes from the brain cells. Just as the juice in the fruit jar contains sugar, salt, and spices, the cerebrospi-nal fluid contains glucose (sugar), proteins, and other impor-tant chemicals and nutrients. Most of the spinal fluid is found in the four cavities (ventricles) that lie in the middle of the brain. Under normal conditions these cavities are small and slit-like. The fluid flows between these four intercon-nected chambers, down to the base of the brain and through several openings or outlets to the surface of the brain where it bathes the brain surface and is finally absorbed (Figure 4). Unlike the fruit, however, the brain is alive and makes its

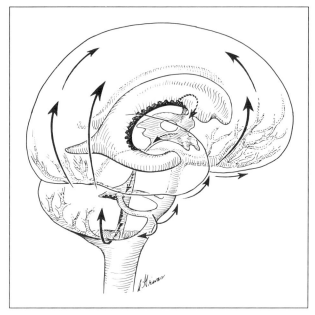

FIGURE 4.
The spinal-fluid pathways in the brain. The flow is from the lateral ventricles (cavities) within the brain, to its base at the back of the head, and then to the brain surface, where it is absorbed.

own fluid in specialized areas called the **choroid plexus**, which lie within the ventricular brain cavities. The average baby needs only a few tablespoons of CSF to protect and bathe its brain. However, much more fluid is produced every day, the excess simply passing onto the brain surface where it is ultimately absorbed into the bloodstream.

It is this "simple" draining process which malfunctions or is obstructed when a baby has an open neural tube defect. Some babies with spina bifida have this CSF obstruction at birth, but most don't develop the problem fully until a number of days have passed. Even when the drainage of the fluid is blocked, the choroid plexus continues to produce CSF. The fluid then begins to accumulate rapidly, which causes pressure to build. Now if this were to happen in the fruit jar, the peaches would first be compressed and then later, as the pressure increased, the jar would eventually explode if it couldn't expand. In a rough comparison, when fluid accumulates within a baby's head, first the brain is gently compressed and then with more pressure it is squeezed. At this point, the head begins to expand as pressure inside builds. Fortunately, the bones in a newborn's skull are still soft and have not yet solidified or fused together. An obvious example of this lack of fusion of a baby's skull is the soft spot on the top of the head (also called the anterior **fontanel**), an area in which the individual skull bones are still far apart. Although the baby's soft flexible skull prevents the head from exploding, there is still a significant possibility for damage when the brain is compressed by the expanding ventricular cavities against the surrounding bony skull (Figure 5).

There are several methods of determining whether a baby is developing hydrocephalus. The easiest involves simply observing the size and shape of the baby's head. In hydrocephalus, there is an enlargement of the head in general, especially in the forehead region. The next step beyond simple observation is to measure the size or circumference of the baby's head. These methods, however, only tell us when the head has begun to expand from pressure within. With modern technology we can now look inside the infant's skull to see if the cavities (ventricles) are enlarging and if they are beginning to compress the brain tissue. A CT or CAT (Computed Tomography) scan uses computer-directed x-rays to survey the brain. For this painless test, the baby lies on a bed inside what looks like an oil drum, while the CT scanner takes cross-sectional pictures of areas of the brain. These images are processed by a computer and specific parts of the brain can be identified. It is somewhat like looking at a loaf of bread one slice at a time. Although it takes special training for the radiologist, neurosurgeon, and neurologist to interpret CT scans, some of the extreme changes in hydrocephalus are quite obvious to even casual examination and can be seen in Figures 5 and 6. Figure 6 represents a normal CT

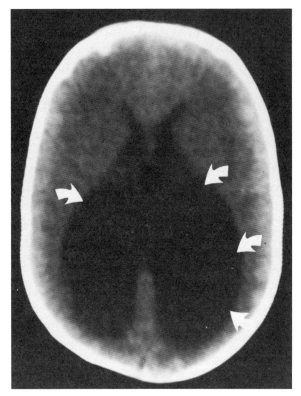

FIGURE 5.
A typical cross-sectional head CT scan of a child with hydrocephalus. Note
the enlarged ventricles (blackened area outlined with arrows) compressing
the brain against the skull (the white-ovoid rim).

scan, with the gray area representing the healthy brain tissue
and the black butterfly-shaped spaces in the middle of the
brain, the normal cavities or ventricles. As noted, Figure 5 is
a CT picture of the brain of a child with a significant hydrocephalus. There is only a thin rim of gray because the normal
brain tissue is being compressed against the skull by the
expanded ventricles.

Another simple imaging technique that can be used to

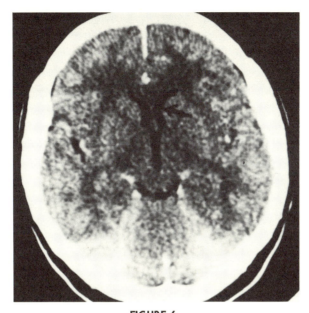

FIGURE 6.
A brain CT scan of a normal infant. Note the small slit-like ventricles, in contrast to those in Figure 5.

complement CAT scanning is ultrasound. Ultrasound uses painless and silent high-frequency sound waves that are reflected back to construct pictures. The technology is similar to that used in SONAR for submarines, with the sound waves traveling through and reflected back from fluid and soft tissue. Figure 7 is an ultrasound picture of a small baby's brain, providing a side view of an enlarged ventricle. Since the sound waves have difficulty passing through bone, ultrasound currently cannot be used in older children and can be used to evaluate hydrocephalus only when there is a bony window in the baby's skull such as the soft spot.

After one or more of the methods described above has shown that the baby has hydrocephalus, decisions about how best to treat the child need to be considered. The pri-

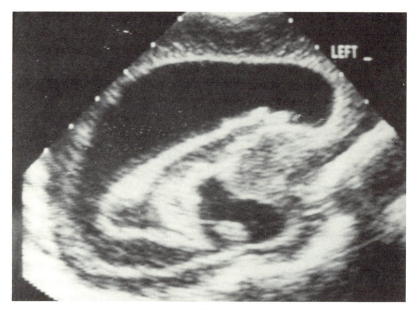

FIGURE 7.
An ultrasound (side) view of a baby's brain. Note the enlarged ventricle (comma-shaped black area).

mary goal of all treatment methods is to relieve the effect of the expanded ventricles and fluid pressure compressing and stretching the surrounding brain tissue.

Among the medical or nonsurgical measures for treatment of hydrocephalus are several drugs that have been used with limited success. They decrease the amount of CSF being made or increase its absorption. Usually these drugs work only for the more mild cases of hydrocephalus and are not generally successful when the hydrocephalus is of the type associated with myelodysplasia, often referred to as obstructive hydrocephalus.

The most common definitive treatment for hydrocephalus involves the surgical placement of a device for diverting or shunting the CSF from the enlarged ventricles. This very narrow soft tube, commonly referred to as a **shunt**, is placed in one of the ventricular cavities of the brain. It allows relief of the CSF pressure and draining of the extra fluid through the tubing under the skin into another body cavity. Shunts are usually made of a soft non-reactive plastic (silastic). They look and feel like a piece of cooked spaghetti and have an inner opening as thin as pencil lead (Figure 8). One end of the shunt tubing is placed into one of the brain cavities (ventricles) by the neurosurgeon through an incision in the scalp and a small hole in the skull. This portion of the shunt system is referred to as the **ventricular** catheter. A patch of the baby's hair needs to be shaved before surgery. This shaved area is usually the most obvious external sign that the baby has been shunted. The other end of the tube passes beneath the scalp behind the ear and then under the skin of the neck to another part of the body where the fluid can be easily absorbed. The most common site is across the chest and into the peritoneal or abdominal cavity, where it remains outside the cavities of the stomach and intestine. This portion of the shunt is referred to as the peritoneal catheter. A shunt of this type going to the baby's stomach is called a V-P or ventriculo-peritoneal shunt. Another less common type of shunt goes into the jugular vein in the neck and then into the first chamber (atrium) of the heart, where the fluid is drained away in the bloodstream. This is referred to as a ventriculo-atrial, or V-A, shunt.

Shunts have undergone considerable change and refinement since they were first utilized some three decades ago. One important part of the upper portion of the shunt is the valve. In most shunts, the valve is contained in an enlarged area of the tubing (Figure 8). It serves two important functions. The first is to be certain that the fluid flows in only one direction through the shunt, since it is important that the extra CSF goes out of the ventricles and that nothing else sneaks in. The other function of the valve is to ensure that the excess pressure and fluid are released, but that some of the CSF stays behind. Remember the example of the fruit jar. Some minimal fluid and fluid pressure are essential to cushion and keep the brain protected.

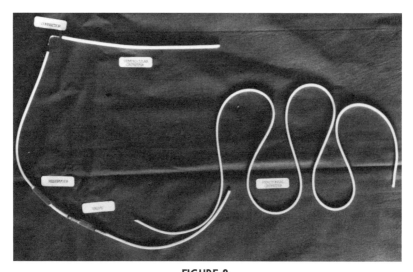

FIGURE 8.
A typical shunt system for treating hydrocephalus. Note the several components: ventricular catheter, reservoir, valve, and peritoneal (abdominal) catheter.

Another important part of the upper shunt is the reservoir. This blister or enlargement of the shunt tubing (usually located in the system just before the valve), allows the surgeon to evaluate the shunt in the future in case of suspected infection or blockage of the shunt. This is accomplished by a so-called shunt tap or shunt aspiration. This minor procedure is generally carried out when there is some question of shunt malfunction or infection. It permits the surgeon to measure the CSF pressure, sample fluid for analysis, and culture for infection, but also to flush the system, in an attempt to relieve a minor blockage problem.

The final point in shunt technology is at the peritoneal end. As a baby grows, the distance between the head and stomach increases. To prevent the baby from rapidly outgrowing the shunt, extra tubing is inserted into the peritoneal cavity at the time the shunt is initially inserted. As the baby grows, the tubing slowly pulls out of the abdominal cavity, but with this extra length its end remains within the cavity for many months.

When a baby returns to the intensive-care nursery after the shunting operation, some changes may already be obvious. The baby's head may be smaller, the skin over the fontanel (soft spot) may be less tightly stretched, and the baby may seem less irritable and more alert. Shunt surgery usually takes less time than the operation to close the baby's back. The effectiveness of a shunt can be seen very clearly on before and after CT scans of the brain or before and after ultrasound studies of the head.

A shunt is an effective treatment for hydrocephalus as long as it is in place. But it can stop working. These malfunctions are generally caused when the tubing becomes plugged or when there is infection around the shunt. The cells and protein that float in the spinal fluid can easily clog the apparatus. When this happens, the signs and symptoms of hydrocephalus reappear. These are often more dramatic in an older baby or child than in a newborn, since the skull is now less flexible and pressure can build more quickly. In addition, as can be seen in Table 1, the problem can be confused with a variety of illnesses present in any baby or child. That's why it is important for any child with a shunt to see a physician when he or she seems sick or is not behaving normally. As parents come to know their child well, they often become expert at distinguishing normal baby fussiness from shunt malfunction. Shunt problems occur most frequently in infancy or early childhood. There seem to be fewer difficulties with older children or adults.

If a shunt is malfunctioning, it may need to be replaced. Sometimes just the ventricular end needs to be changed; at other times the peritoneal catheter or valve and, in some cases, the whole apparatus needs to be removed and replaced. Usually only a few days of hospitalization are required. Some children never have shunt problems, while others experience multiple malfunctions or other difficulties.

Aside from observation, children with shunts usually need no special protection or care. They can be held, jiggled, and

Table 1. Some Signs and Symptoms of Shunt Problems

Babies	Toddlers	Children	Adults
	Headaches	Headaches	Headaches
Fussiness/ Irritability	Crankiness/ Irritability	Crabbiness	Personality change
Vomiting	Vomiting	Vomiting	Vomiting
Bulging soft spot (fontanel)		School problems	Lethargy
Expanding head size (especially in the forehead)		Difficulty with balance or coordination	Difficulty with balance or coordination
Change in eating patterns			
Lethargy	Lethargy	Lethargy	Lethargy
Sleepiness	Sleepiness	Sleepiness	Sleepiness
Eyes gaze downward like a sunset	Visual blurring	Visual blurring	Visual blurring or blind spots
Seizures	Seizures	Seizures	Seizures

tickled. Very small babies with poor head control should not lie continuously on a shunt, since their scalp is thin and a pressure area or sore may develop over the shunt apparatus. As the infant gets older and gains head control, this becomes less of a worry. When considering activities for older children and teenagers, most neurosurgeons recommend that contact sports be avoided. Usually a common-sense approach applies, trying to avoid activities where there is a likelihood of significant head bumps or trauma. Finally, since the shunt represents an implanted foreign body subject to infection, many doctors suggest antibiotic prophylaxis at the time of any surgery or major dental work.

As we noted in the beginning, every child, and every person with spina bifida, is different. So is every case of hydrocephalus. The team caring for the child and most particularly the neurosurgeon are the best sources of information for specific questions or concerns.

Orthopedic Problems

As we indicated in our discussion of nerve damage, most children with spina bifida have abnormalities in the nerves leading to their legs. The motor and sensory (moving and feeling) deficits that result vary greatly, depending on the extent to which the child's spinal cord is impaired. Because of these variations, it is impossible to generalize about the orthopedic problems children with spina bifida may experience. We'll begin by introducing the professionals who can provide families with advice about and treatment for the bone, muscle, and joint problems associated with spina bifida.

After hearing that their baby has spina bifida, parents usually ask, "Will our baby be able to walk?" The most honest answer at this point is frequently: "It's too soon to tell, we'll have to wait and see." As noted earlier, there are many limitations on the muscle and nerve testing that can be done on a baby. Probably a more appropriate question is, "Will our child be able to get around?" The answer is almost always, "Yes."

Along the way to mobility, there are many different professionals, both in the hospital and in the community, who can assist the child and the family. The **orthopedist** or **orthopedic surgeon**, commonly referred to as a "bone doctor," is one of the key individuals in these matters. It is interesting to go back to the Greek roots of the word — "orthos" for straight and "paedia" for child — to see that orthopedics has a lot to offer the child with spina bifida. The **physiatrist**, a doctor who specializes in physical medicine and rehabilitation, can often contribute to the nonsurgical care of the bones, muscles, and joints of a child with spina bifida. Physical therapists work with physicians to evaluate and treat motor problems, and **orthotists** make the braces which are so often essential for mobility.

Some babies with spina bifida have very obvious deformities of their legs and feet, which are evident at birth. These

abnormalities can best be understood by becoming acquainted with how muscles function. They are the servants
of the nerves, doing the work of moving body parts, joints,
and limbs. Skeletal muscles move only on command of their
masters, the nerves. A muscle is somewhat like a rubber
band that stretches out and springs back. Each bone and
joint is controlled by several different muscles which in turn
are governed by nerves. One muscle or group of muscles
may be responsible for bending a joint; another may be
responsible for straightening it out. In most situations, the
two muscle groups are in balance; the strength of the two
groups is equal so that the limb or joint is in a normal or neu-
tral position. However, with the nerve damage typical in
spina bifida, one muscle may end up functioning normally
while its opposing partner is paralyzed. This results in a
deformed or bent joint or limb. These changes in the shape
of the bones and joints can develop even in the fetus. The
result is an unopposed muscle pull at a joint producing a
deformity which may be quite apparent even in the delivery
room.

There are many different modes of treatment for the
abnormalities present at birth and those that may develop
later. It is often confusing to parents when they hear several
different opinions or when they see their child receiving
treatment different from the treatment being given another
child who seems to have the same problem. Although some
of the differences in treatment reflect differences between
children, others reflect an individual physician's or surgeon's preference. Often these different approaches in treatment reflect the fact that many of these situations have no
black or white, no right or wrong answers. Each treatment
has its own benefits and risks and its own chances of success
and failure. Moreover, doctors are constantly learning about
the long-term effects of treatment and at the same time
developing new methods. In this book we cannot identify a
right or a wrong way to treat a particular child with his or her
own unique difficulties. What we can do is to introduce some

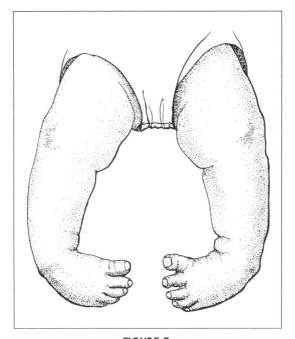

FIGURE 9.
A clubfoot deformity in a small baby. Note the downward and inward positioning of the feet.

of the common orthopedic problems and describe, in general terms, some of the treatments available.

Club Foot

One of the most common orthopedic problems seen in children with spina bifida and partial paralysis of the lower extremities is a condition referred to as a club foot. **Talipes equinovarus** is the medical term for this condition in which one or both feet point down and inward (Figure 9). This condition is often treated with tiny casts that are put on the baby's feet to push them gradually up and outward. The casts are usually changed every week or so, with each new

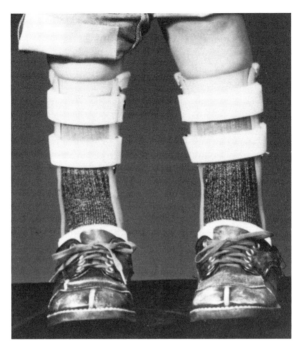

FIGURE 10.
Standard ankle-foot orthoses (AFO) for bracing the ankles.

cast designed to nudge the foot into a more normal position. This succession of plaster casts is called serial casting. Even when the baby is being treated, it is often not clear whether he or she will be able to walk later. In any case, correcting the club foot deformity will make walking easier, and it will be easier to fit shoes. Sometimes after a few weeks or months, the child's feet will have been molded into a more normal position. At this point, the orthopedist may ask the orthotist to construct small braces to maintain the baby's feet in a normal position as further growth occurs (Figure 10). Many brace shops now construct these braces or orthoses from polypropylene, a light-weight plastic material. This provides the same amount of support as the more traditional metal and leather braces, but it is light enough and thin enough to fit inside baby booties or even sneakers as the child grows older. As the child outgrows the braces, the continued need for them is re-evaluated.

Sometimes there is a limit to the amount of correction that can be done through serial casting, and the orthopedist will often then suggest surgery to further correct the club foot deformity. In this situation, a minor operation releases the contracted soft tissues at the heel cord, a "heel cord release." If indicated, it may be done even before the baby's first birthday. After the major tendon to the heel bone is divided, the foot can then slip upward into a more normal position. After surgery, casts are often applied for a number of weeks to maintain the feet in the desired position. Braces are often fitted afterward.

If serial casting and soft tissue releases fail to leave the foot in a normal position, other operations can be considered. These procedures are more extensive and involve realigning and reforming the bones in the foot and heel. They are often delayed until the child is at least one year old.

Other Deformities

Beside club feet, there are other rigid deformities evident at birth in a child with spina bifida. For example, in an infant with a high lumbar sensory and motor level lesion, the only muscle groups functioning in the lower extremities may be those that control hip flection or bending. Here the muscles opposing hip flection are paralyzed. As a consequence, the hips are held in a flexed or bent position. Other deformities may produce contractures (frozen or stiff joints) at the knees. Again these develop because the muscles pulling in one direction may be working, but the muscles designed to balance the joint and to tug back in the opposite direction may not be getting the nerve messages to tell them to work. The joint then begins to grow like a plant that gets light on only one side. If this unequal stimulation continues, the contracture becomes permanent and may be severe enough to cause the joint to actually dislocate (**subluxation**). This occurs most frequently at the hip. In this situation, special splints may be used, designed to maintain the hip joint in a position where the dislocation has been corrected.

If a joint is fixed or always held in the same position, it will hinder a child's ability to move about. Physical therapists can do a series of exercises on contracted joints called range of motion exercises. These are referred to as active range of motion exercises if the child can help or assist in the movement and passive range of motion exercises if all the muscles at the joint are paralyzed. These maneuvers ensure that the joints have a full range of motion, because they are moved in all directions. Parents can learn to move the baby's joints to carry out range of motion exercises. They may do this when the baby is being bathed and dressed or even with each diaper change. Keeping the baby's limbs supple can go a long way toward preventing serious problems. Parents may also be instructed in sleeping positions that will prevent joint dislocation or deformity and discourage contractures from becoming permanent.

Developing Motor Skills

Babies acquire skills in a step-by-step fashion. We're all familiar with the saying, "You have to walk, before you can learn to run." Babies need to sit before they can crawl and crawl before they can walk. Babies with spina bifida go through a similar process. At some steps they need extra encouragement, and at other points an alternative may need to be substituted. This early learning process may be interrupted or even set back when an infant is ill. The first year for a baby with spina bifida may be complicated by numerous trips to the hospital for treatment of shunt malfunction, for serial casting, and for other surgery. These can temporarily interfere with early learning and development.

Early learning can be aided by enrolling the baby in an infant stimulation program. Many cities and localities now have these programs which are designed to give a boost to handicapped children from the time they first leave the hospital. Physical therapists, public health nurses, and social workers can often assist parents in contacting these programs. Very young children often receive help at home, while toddlers and older children may go to a center for an opportunity to interact with other children, as well as with their teachers and therapists. These early education programs are designed to provide support to parents who are ultimately their baby's most important teachers. There are many different professionals involved with infant stimulation programs. Not every discipline may be represented or required at each center, but often there is the option for consultation. The staff may include a physical therapist, an occupational therapist, a speech and language clinician, a special education teacher, a parent educator, and an infant teacher, among others.

One of the first motor skills an infant acquires is head control. The baby is then able to hold its head up and turn and maintain it in a particular position. This skill may be more difficult to achieve when a baby has a large head owing to hydrocephalus. The next milestone in acquiring gross motor skills (a movement controlled by large muscle groups) is rolling over. A baby with spina bifida may have trouble with this movement because of weakness or paralysis in the lower extremities. Sitting can also be a little more difficult for youngsters with spina bifida. However, like the other skills we've discussed, it can be mastered by almost all children with spina bifida. Although these babies may not follow the time tables of other infants, they will follow the same sequences. Like all of us, children with spina bifida benefit from encouragement and praise. Therapists at the hospital or in an infant stimulation program often have suggestions which help the child attain these skills.

Ambulation and Getting Around

There are many means of locomotion. Not all children will be able to achieve the same skill level. There are, however, also many substitutes. Once again it is well to mention that not every child will meet every goal. Perhaps it would be useful here to stop for a moment to think about what end points we're trying to attain when we move around.

There's long-distance travel, such as marathon running and "walking 20 miles to school." Some motion, such as our passion for cross-country skiing and walking in the country, is recreational. We walk through our communities to go shopping or dash from the office copier to a desk, and we move a lot within our own homes to do housework, eat meals, or change the television channel. Finally, we move very short distances in and out of the bathtub, and in and out of our beds. In the course of these activities, we learn more about our environment, interact with others, earn a living, and perform tasks of daily life. When considering the best way for a child with spina bifida to get around, we must consider not only the child's physical abilities, but also where the youngster is going and why.

The first method that infants use to scoot around is crawling on their abdomen (tummy or belly crawling). In this activity, they use their arms to pull themselves ahead. Most kids rapidly begin to use their legs for extra propulsion. Then they get up on their knees and truly begin to crawl. Children with spina bifida can be great tummy crawlers. However, without the extra boost from their legs, it may be difficult for them to go beyond this stage. Some kids get around well enough to do all the exploring, learning, trouble-making, and getting into cabinets that this developmental stage requires. Others need some equipment to speed them along. A crawling board with casters (either home-made or purchased) adds momentum and assists arm and hand motions. Some children can't generate enough power at these early stages with their arms, and they do better with a type of caster cart (Figure 11). Here the child sits in a bucket seat and spins the back wheels of this low-slung cart while checking out the environment and keeping up with playmates and the puppy.

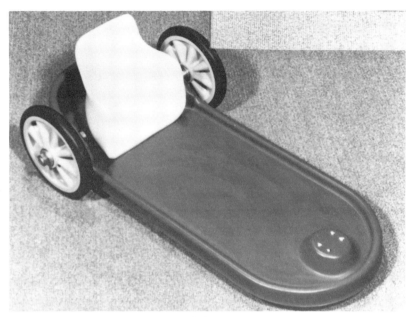

FIGURE 11.
A caster cart, which increases the mobility of a small child whose legs have impaired motor function.

As children get older, they generally move up in the world. First they hang onto furniture, then they begin to travel along its edges, and finally they let go and begin to toddle independently. Standing up and walking independently are very difficult for some children with spina bifida and impossible for others. However, children can be helped to stand by several different devices, such as a standing frame, a crutchless standing orthosis, or a tilt table. These aids will allow the child to "see what the big kids do," develop upper trunk muscles, improve balance, and encourage better circulation and bone growth in the legs.

Some children will pull up along furniture just fine, but as they try to walk, their ankles will appear to give way. In this situation, joints can be stabilized by the use of short leg braces or ankle foot orthoses (AFOs), which come up to mid-calf.

For a child with a more significant paralysis in the legs— for example a toddler whose neurological lesion is above L-5—more help is usually required for walking. In this situation, long leg braces, also called knee-ankle-foot orthoses (KAFOs), may be used. Sometimes a pelvic band to support the waist may provide further assistance. A walker or crutches may also be used to help gain assistance (recruitment) from the child's upper body strength for walking. Just as there are many different styles of braces, there are many kinds of walkers and crutches and various methods for using each one. The therapists and doctors working with each child will design an individualized program using these mobility aids to complement a child's strength and skills.

It can require a lot of time and skill for a child with spina bifida to master these alternative modes of getting around. It is important that the youngster not miss too many of the important parts of growing up along the way. Although a child may be walking well with braces and a walker at school, he or she may not have the endurance and speed necessary to see every animal on a trip to the zoo. At these times, a big stroller or a wheelchair may come in handy. Young children enjoy spending time outside with their friends. Kids with spina bifida may have a hard time keeping up on foot, but a hand-driven tricycle may be the envy of the neighborhood.

As a child spends more time upright, in braces and learning to walk, it may become obvious that certain orthopedic abnormalities are interfering with the process. Surgical correction of these problems may improve ambulation.

Spinal Deformities

One additional area that can cause a problem for children with spina bifida is the spine, or more precisely the vertebrae. To best understand spinal disorders in spina bifida there are two more words to add to your vocabulary, **kyph-osis** and **scoliosis**. Both of these terms refer to a curvature of the spine. With kyphosis, the spine is bent or curved forward. If severe enough, it produces a hump on the back, which in some instances may be quite visible. In scoliosis, the curvature is to the side and there may be some twisting. Children with spina bifida are more vulnerable to these problems because of malformed vertebrae in the spine and because of weakened or paralyzed muscles controlling spinal movements. If the child has a large myelomeningocele involving the area up to the mid-back (thoracic area), a kyphosis may even be present at birth, making repair and closure of the myelomeningocele quite difficult. If a kyphosis is severe, it can even interfere with the child's ability to sit. In this case, surgical correction and fusion by an orthopedic surgeon may be desirable.

In less serious cases, a spinal curvature may slowly develop at a later age. This happens because when the muscles along the spine are weak or paralyzed, it is difficult for the spine to grow straight. This crookedness (scoliosis) is often exaggerated during the growth spurts of late childhood and early adolescence. If the orthopedist notes that a scoliosis is progressing, a brace or plastic body jacket may be recommended to remind the spine to grow straight. If the curvature worsens, surgery may again be necessary to halt the progression of the curvature and prevent further deformity. In a youngster with spina bifida, severe scoliosis can interfere not only with the ability to get around, but also with his or her overall health.

Urological and Bladder Problems

Although it is relatively easy to understand how the sac on the back is related to lower limb paralysis and indirectly associated with hydrocephalus, it is not always immediately obvious why the bladder and kidneys can also be affected by a myelomeningocele. Problems in bladder sensation and motor control are common in spina bifida. The bladder has sensation and its wall is primarily muscular. The nerves controlling the bladder come out of the lowest sacral (S2-S5) portion of the spinal cord, even further down than the nerves to the feet (Figure 3). As a consequence, nearly all individuals with myelodysplasia have some degree of bladder nerve involvement, even in cases where the feet and ankles are minimally involved. **Urologists** are the doctors who are experts in treating conditions of the bladder and the rest of the urinary tract.

All of the body's blood passes through the kidneys many times a day. In the adult, these two potato-sized and bean-shaped organs lie deeply seated in the mid back and are very sophisticated filters designed to remove extra water, waste products, and harmful substances from the body (Figure 12). The extra water and its waste products (urine) filtered out of the blood by the kidneys then flow downward toward the pelvis through a small spaghetti-like tube (**ureter**) from each kidney to the bladder, where it is stored until it is emptied (Figure 12). When the bladder is full, sensory nerves send messages back to the spinal cord, where a reflex reaction occurs through the bladder motor nerves, telling the muscles of the bladder wall to contract and to empty the bladder by pushing the urine out through the **urethra**. The urethra is the short tube-like passageway from the bladder to the body surface. There are also valves made of muscle called **sphincters** along the urethra. These sphincters allow the neurologically mature individual to choose when to urinate.

When a child has spina bifida, the sensory and motor nerves to the bladder are impaired, so it is difficult for the child to know when the bladder is full, and it is difficult for the bladder to empty appropriately, either reflexively or voluntarily. Since no baby has good voluntary sphincter control, the newborn with a neural tube defect is no different from any other infant in needing diapers. However, despite this lack of difference in bladder control, many infants with spina bifida have weak bladder muscles and as a result are

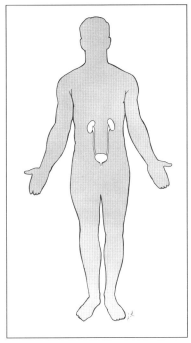

FIGURE 12.

The urinary system. The kidneys are deep in the back, with ureters (tube-like structures) connecting the kidneys to the bladder located just behind the pubic bone.

unable to empty their bladder completely. Having old urine lingering in the bladder can create a health problem, since stagnant urine can result in a chronic infection. Moreover, this leftover infected urine can travel back up the ureters (**reflux**) into the kidneys. Ultimately, this infected urinary reflux can cause kidney infections and finally kidney damage. On occasion it may be severe and can result in kidney or renal failure. Before the significance of preventing reflux was understood, many children with spina bifida died of kidney damage and renal failure.

When a newborn's muscles are not strong enough to empty its bladder, the **Crede maneuver** may be used to assist it to empty more completely. Initially, the nurses begin this maneuver, in which they push down on the lower tummy wall to apply pressure over the bladder. Parents may also learn this technique. Creding is not as popular as it once was because of the observation that while most of the urine is eliminated, some can unfortunately be forced up or refluxed into the kidneys.

Many tests can be done during infancy and beyond to assess the health and functioning of the urinary tract. It is essential that a child with spina bifida see a urologist familiar with his or her condition on a regular basis. Reflux and early signs of kidney damage may not be obvious without proper urologic testing.

The simplest of tests involves observation of the baby to see if voiding is done in a stream or if there is constant urinary dribbling. Other tests can show if the kidney is allowing normal amounts of chemicals such as sodium and potassium to circulate in the bloodstream. Blood tests for levels of **blood urea nitrogen** (BUN) or **creatinine** also indicate how well the urinary system is functioning, since these waste chemicals build up if the bladder and kidneys are not working appropriately.

Urine can also be studied (urinalysis) to make sure that chemicals are being eliminated in the proper concentration. A urinalysis will also tell if there is blood or other inappropriate substances in the urine. In addition, children with spina bifida may need frequent urine cultures to check for signs of infection. As noted, this is a particularly troublesome problem in some patients. Sometimes the urine can be collected by placing a small bag over the little boy's penis or little girl's bottom (**perineum**). At other times catheterization may be necessary. In this procedure, a catheter (a soft thin rubber or pliable plastic tube) is slipped up the urethra into the bladder, to allow for collection of urine without contamination by the bacteria (germs) from the skin surface.

There are other tests to evaluate the structure and function of the urinary tract. Ultrasound can be used to visualize the bladder and kidneys to be certain they are in the proper location and of appropriate size. This is often one of the first urological studies done on a newborn. In addition, x-ray testing of the kidneys (**intravenous pyelograms** or IVPs) is frequently done on a regular basis. In this test, an iodine-containing dye is slowly injected into a vein (usually in front of the elbow). It is then carried by the bloodstream to the kidneys where it is collected, concentrated, and eliminated in the urine. Since the iodine in the dye is visible on x-ray, subsequent x-rays are taken to see the size and shape of the kidneys and ureters as they work to eliminate this dye. Occasionally, some individuals are allergic to the iodine. If a child has an allergic reaction, it is important that this information be put in a prominent place on the medical record.

Other tests can be done to assess the bladder at work such as a **voiding cystourethrogram** (VCUG) or **cystoscopy**. With these tests, the urologist actually looks into the bladder to observe its appearance and function.

If reflux is severe during infancy, the urologist may recommend a **vesicostomy**. During this operation, an opening is made from the bladder out through the abdominal wall, allowing urine to drain directly into the diaper. Most babies do not need this temporary procedure and do quite well in diapers, as do other children their age. It should be noted that children who never have a dry diaper and are constantly dribbling are more prone to diaper rashes and skin irritation. In this case, extra attention is in order. Parents may also be told to give young children extra liquids to drink in order to dilute the urine, but generally at this early age the urinary tract usually requires little extra attention.

As infants mature, their muscle tone and neurological control improve and they are ready for potty training. In view of the frequency of bladder dysfunction in spina bifida, it is only the rare child with myelodysplasia who can master this skill without some special help. As peers and playmates get older, the child with nerve damage may be embarrassed to still be in diapers. In many cases, intermittent catheterization may provide a solution. This procedure involves putting a catheter into the bladder several times per day, with the goals of preventing residual urine buildup and reflux, and keeping the child dry. Until recently, catheterization was done only in a medical setting under sterile conditions, chiefly because of the fear of causing a urinary tract infection. However, studies have shown that when done properly and cleanly by parents, a school nurse, an aide, and eventually by the child, inserting a catheter on a regular basis does not result in extra infection. Finally, other maneuvers or medications are sometimes suggested to help the child remain completely dry between trips to the bathroom for catheterization.

There was a period of time several years ago, after the harm of reflux was understood and before the acceptance of intermittent catheterization, when most young people had a urinary diversion operation. In this procedure, a piece of the small intestine was used to create a permanent channel (**ileostomy**) for urine to flow from the ureters to outside the abdominal wall and into a bag. Ileostomies are still done occasionally, when other means of preventing reflux fail. These ileal diversions never achieved great popularity, and some young adults are now returning to their urologists asking for reimplantation of the ureters into their normal location in the bladder wall.

A new development, the artifical sphincter for the management of incontinence, is now being tested and evaluated. An inflatable cuff is surgically implanted and surrounds the urethra, just below the bladder neck, in an attempt to prevent incontinence and dribbling. When the person wishes to void, a control bag connected to the cuff and implanted in the child's bottom is activated. Like any new technological device, early models had many flaws, some of which are being corrected. Owing to differences in male and female anatomy, the artificial sphincter is more successful for males.

Bowel Control Problems

The nerves controlling the sphincter of the rectum are also

frequently affected when a child has myelodysplasia. Practically, the rectal sphincter muscles are most easily and quickly checked by slipping a finger into the anal opening, to determine if there is any muscle tone or tightness. When there is weakness or paralysis, stool passes into the diaper whenever it arrives from the colon, in much the same way that urine dribbles out from the bladder. Luckily there is no equivalent of reflux as far as the bowel is concerned, so in this sense there are no serious health risks to the baby.

As a toddler grows older, however, it is less socially acceptable to frequently have a dirty diaper. The child with spina bifida may not have the sensation of a full rectum, so will not have the urge for a bowel movement, making toilet and bowel training difficult. However, most individuals are able to establish a regular schedule for bowel movements and emptying the rectum, and by following this routine can minimize accidents. A temporary illness with diarrhea can be a difficult time. Often modifying the diet with high fiber foods and extra liquids makes this approach work better. Physiatrists, pediatricians, and nurses who work with children with spina bifida are good resources for development of an effective bowel program.

Problems with Skin Sensation

From our first description of the nerve damage associated with myelodysplasia, we've stressed that both the moving (motor or muscle) and feeling (sensory, i.e., touch, pain, temperature) nerves are affected (Figure 2). Although the disability associated with impaired motor nerves is the most obvious to the casual observer, sensory nerve impairment is equally important and can be responsible for chronic health problems. Individuals with normal skin sensation have an immediate and reflexive response to painful contact. If you put your hand on a hot stove or step on a tack, you will wince and move away so quickly that you are not even aware of the decision you've made. When a person has sensory nerve impairment, as with spina bifida, this sort of response is diminished or even absent in the area where the nerves are damaged.

A hot stove or a rusty nail are dramatic examples of this decreased response. However, it is usually constant small irritants and injuries that cause problems for a person with spina bifida. When a person with intact sensation wears shoes that are too tight, the nerves in the feet send up messages of pain. The person may then change positions, wiggle the toes, or even take off the shoes. If the shoes are not changed soon enough, a blister may develop. If the foot is sore enough, it is unlikely the individual will put on the same shoe the next day. A person with spina bifida may feel little or even no discomfort, so the foot position won't be changed, the shoe won't be taken off, and it may even be worn again the next day because it doesn't hurt! The blister can become further irritated and can then enlarge and extend deeper into the tissues, causing a pressure sore.

Pressure Sores and Decubitus Ulcers

Pressure sores are potentially serious health concerns. At times they can become infected, and they can actually burrow into the underlying tissues (**decubitus ulcer**), even to the point where the underlying bone becomes involved. If the problem gets out of control, the resultant infection can spread to an even larger area and possibly throughout the body. If not properly treated, a grave illness is then possible. Therapy is most successful and complications are minimized when treatment is undertaken in the early stages, while the problem is still minor. Besides an alteration in or a lack of skin sensation, there are other contributing factors associated with spina bifida that predispose the individual to pressure sores. If there are contractures or if limbs are deformed or not properly aligned, weight may rest on areas or body parts less protected and less able to handle the load. In addition, circulation to the legs may be lessened, especially if

Table 2.
Precautions for Skin with Diminished Sensation

1. Do not stay in the same position for a long time. People in wheelchairs need to shift frequently and do wheelchair push-ups.

2. Do not sleep or doze on a hard surface.

3. Smooth out wrinkles in stockings before putting on shoes or braces.

4. *Always* check skin when putting on and taking off shoes and braces.

5. Reddened skin areas should cause immediate concern. Some assistance in out of sight areas may be necessary.

6. Cover legs when a child or infant is crawling across the floor.

7. Avoid hot bathtub water; luke-warm water is a must.

8. Consider lowering the temperature on the hot water heater.

9. Don't stay too close to a radiator, fireplace, or stove.

10. Don't sit on a car seat heated by the sun; consider a sheepskin.

11. Proper shoe size and an appropriate fit are imperative.

12. Always keep the skin dry and clean. For babies, frequent diaper changes are essential.

they are not actively used, so the blood flow needed to maintain healthy tissues and skin is not maintained. Finally, areas that are always moist are also more vulnerable to skin breakdown. Table 2 outlines many of the "do's and don't's" concerning skin care and prevention of pressure sores.

The treatment of serious pressure sores can be a lengthy and laborious task requiring the cooperation of the patient, family, and medical staff. The first step is to remove and avoid any further pressure from the affected area. In addition, other irritants need to be kept clear of the region. If there's a sore on the foot, the person may need to remove the brace or shoe. If the sore is on the buttocks, prolonged sitting, especially in a wheelchair, must be curtailed or at times totally avoided. Obviously these measures may temporarily interfere with an individual's ability to get around. If a pressure sore is small, medications may be directly applied. Larger infected areas may require treatment with antibiotics, at times in the hospital. Some large decubitus wounds may even require surgical **debridement** (clean-up), repair, and possibly even skin grafting.

Given the serious nature of pressure sores, it is obvious that an ounce of prevention is worth much more than a pound of cure. There are many precautions that when faithfully observed are very effective in reducing the risk of pressure sores. If a sore does develop, the earlier that treatment is initiated, the more likely it is to be successful. Pressure sores are more common during adolescence and young adulthood than during childhood. However, the precautions listed in Table 2 are best learned early in life.

Other Health Problems

We have now discussed the problems that affect most children with spina bifida. Other more general childhood problems may also develop. Many ordinary conditions such as colds, chicken pox, or allergies are just as common in children with neural tube defects as they are in other children. And most of the time these conditions can be managed in the same way for all children. Some physicians may not have had a great deal of experience with spina bifida and its problems, and may consult an expert to see if a special approach is needed for these ordinary matters.

Other conditions may develop, and it may not be clear if they are related to spina bifida and any of its associated problems; if it's a complication of treatment the person may be currently undergoing; or if it's a totally unrelated issue. Headache is a good example of such a problem and one that can be especially difficult to evaluate in a person with spina bifida. You will recall that in an earlier section we listed headache as a sign of shunt failure in the child with hydrocephalus. However, headaches can also be caused by eye strain, the flu, tension, or simply not wanting to go to school. Sometimes it takes a bit of persistence and clever medical and family detective work to sort out these problems.

In addition to general medical problems affecting everyone, there are other conditions that are more common among individuals with spina bifida. Not every child with spina bifida will develop all or even any of these conditions. Nor does this discussion include all potential difficulties and problems.

Weight and Overeating

Obesity can be a serious problem for individuals with spina bifida. Being heavy can make it much more difficult to get around. For the child with spina bifida, an extra 20 pounds may make the difference between being able to manage well on crutches and being in a wheelchair. Obesity can also make a person more vulnerable to pressure sores. Once a person with spina bifida is overweight, it may be very difficult to lose those extra pounds, especially because he or she may have a less active lifestyle. While cutting down on calories is possible, it may be difficult to exercise enough to contribute to weight reduction. Once again, it is easier to prevent the problem than to cure it. Children and adolescents may eat out of boredom and inactivity, with disastrous effects on the waistline. Establishing a healthy low-calorie diet early in life is beneficial, and although it is easier said than done, for purposes of good health maintenance the cycle of overeating and excess weight needs to be broken early.

Disturbances in Height

At the other side of the growth spectrum are disturbances in height. Short stature is common in children with spina bifida. The cause of this difficulty is not well understood, nor is there agreement on a treatment approach. Some growth lag is certainly due to the bony abnormalities in the vertebral column. For example, if scoliosis develops—with the spine curving off to the side—height will not increase as much as expected. In addition, if the curvature is severe enough to require a spinal fusion, in the future there will be no further growth in the fused spinal segments. However, the very short stature of some children with spina bifida exceeds what might be expected solely from a disturbance of spinal growth. **Pediatric endocrinologists**, who specialize in growth disorders of childhood, may be consulted when there is concern about a child's height. These physicians are skilled in discovering causes of delay in physical development, including short stature. Parents and children often raise questions about treatment with substances such as growth hormone to help the child become taller. Hormone treatment is still controversial, and these decisions must be made on an individual basis. It is also helpful to consider that it is not always advantageous for an individual with a physical disability to be bigger or, for that matter, taller. Questions that need to be asked include: "Will growing faster increase scoliosis?" and "Will it be easier or more difficult to get around if I'm taller?"

Seizures and Epilepsy

Another problem that children with spina bifida are more likely to develop is seizures. A seizure represents a disturbance in the normal pattern of electrical activity within the brain. In a seizure, the brain's normal cyclical and rhythmic electrical activity becomes abnormal and uncontrolled. Seizures used to be called convulsions or fits. When a person has had several or many seizures, a diagnosis of epilepsy is made. When the electrical activity of the brain is abnormal, there can be a variety of different external manifestations. The child's whole body may jerk rhythmically and go limp, or the eyelids may simply flutter and the child may seem to be in a daze. Neurologists are the specialists who deal most with seizures. In their assessment of a problem, one of the major tools for studying seizures is the **electroencephalo-gram** (EEG). During this test, sticky electrodes are pasted on the child's scalp to measure and record the brain's electrical activity. The EEG machine simultaneously records these rhythmic electrical impulses from a number of brain areas. Squiggly lines from the machine, representing the brain's micro-electrical waves, are drawn on continuously running strips of graph paper. Interpretation of these waves and patterns assists the neurologist in understanding more about the situation, e.g., whether the spells are truly seizures and if so what type and from what area of the brain.

Children with hydrocephalus may have seizures because of shunt malfunction or infection. After the shunt problem is corrected, the seizures frequently disappear, but seizures can also occur even while the shunt is working quite properly. These seizures probably result from a variety of causes, including damage from the hydrocephalus, brain scarring from past infection, irritation around the shunt tube, or abnormal brain tissue arising from an associated birth defect. It is essential that seizures in a child with spina bifida be appropriately and promptly evaluated. If the shunt is malfunctioning, it can be repaired or replaced. If the brain is sending out inappropriate electrical signals resulting in seizures without a specific cause, there are medications which are usually very effective in controlling the problem. If major seizures are not treated, additional brain damage may result.

Visual Problems

Children with spina bifida are also more vulnerable to problems with vision. Nearsightedness is common, as are problems with the balance of the eye muscles resulting in "crossed eyes," referred to medically as **esotropia**. Sometimes surgery is necessary for correction of the problem. For a child whose mobility is impaired, being able to see well is especially important. For this reason, many children with spina bifida need to see an **ophthalmologist** when they are very young and often regularly thereafter. These physicians are specialists in eye problems and will be able to ensure that the child has an optimum window on the world.

Chapter 3
GROWING UP

When considering the impact of a disability, there are two possible approaches: the effects on different body systems and the effects at different ages. Up to this point we have discussed only the impact of spina bifida on organ systems and bodily functions. The following sections are devoted to an age-based approach. Obviously, these two perspectives of the condition are closely inter-twined. For example, the size and location of the sac, and the varying degrees of nerve impairment associated with it, will influence what kind of schooling is most appropriate and will determine the amount of independence possible in adulthood. Similarly, the child's age and stage of develop-ment will influence which medical and therapeutic strategies are used for particular conditions or complications associated with spina bifida.

The Infant and Young Child

As mentioned earlier, the birth of a child with spina bifida comes as a shock to most parents. Usually they have had no warning of a problem, so they have gone through the nine months of pregnancy planning for the arrival of a healthy baby. They have picked out names, purchased a crib, had baby showers, and dreamed of the future. When the baby has a birth defect, many things change. Instead of being able to cuddle their new baby, the baby is whisked away and the parents are asked to consent to surgery! Usually, they have never heard of spina bifida and are now being asked to quickly master a vocabulary that would rival that of many medical students. One of the most difficult situations is when the mother is in one hospital and the baby has been transferred to another. Furthermore, it is difficult for them to get acquainted if the new baby remains hospitalized. Recognizing this difficult situation, many **Newborn Intensive Care Units** (NICUs) can make arrangements for the mother and baby to spend some time together before the baby is discharged. Often the hospital social worker can assist in this matter. Finally, even if everything has gone well, it can be frightening to take home a baby who has had one or more operations and who may need some special treatments and observation. Getting to know the baby, trying to learn about spina bifida and hydrocephalus, and participating in treatment decisions can make this transition easier.

On rare occasions, some young parents are too overwhelmed by their baby's disability to consider taking the infant home. They may feel they cannot be good parents for a child with a handicap, or they may think the baby's problems will make it too difficult to care for their other children. When this is the case, the parents may want to place the baby into foster care or for adoption. Often this is one of the most difficult decisions that loving parents can make. In many areas in the country, there are waiting lists of couples who want to adopt babies with disabilities, including spina bifida. If this is not the situation in a particular region, social workers or social-service agencies can contact their state Spina Bifida Association or, if one does not exist, the Spina Bifida Association of America (SBAA), which runs a National Placement Referral Service.

The Spina Bifida Association is an excellent informational resource for parents. Regional or state SBA chapters can be located by contacting the national SBAA office, asking hospital staff members, or even looking in the telephone directory under spina bifida. The SBAA has a wealth of printed material, and among its many membership services are lists of Spina Bifida Clinics, newsletters, and parent-support groups. (See the appendix for specific information.)

Before leaving the hospital with the baby, parents should be certain they know how to generally care for their child, and they should be familiar with any special treatments that are necessary, how they are done, and if they can be accomplished by mom or dad with ease and comfort. Also, parents should know the danger signs to watch for, who should be called if the baby gets sick, when and where followup appointments are scheduled, and who can provide help in their local community. Finally, as with all infants, a special car seat is needed to keep the baby safe while traveling.

Most experts suggest that children with spina bifida be followed by the staff of a special spina bifida clinic. As we've noted, individuals with spina bifida need the care of a variety of health professionals. The "one-stop shopping" available in spina bifida clinics (commonly referred to as "myelo clinics") makes coordination of appointments easier for families. More important, the health professionals who treat many patients with spina bifida have ready access to the necessary support services for their patients, and, most important, they also have greater experience in the fine points of handling the special needs and problems associated with spina bifida. Before their baby is discharged from the hospital, parents should inquire about the availability of and the possible referral to a spina bifida or myelo clinic. At times, there can be a great distance between the clinic and home. In this situation it is especially important to have a nearby family doctor, pediatrician, or primary-care physician who can help bridge this distance and provide good health care in the local area.

When a child is born with a birth defect, many worries about the future may arise. One of the more troubling concerns is financial. Parents, especially fathers, worry how they will pay medical bills and cover other expenses. For families with medical insurance, it is essential to do whatever clerical tasks are necessary to enroll the baby on the family's policy. It may also be wise to find out what the insurance will pay for and what services are not covered. These inquiries are especially important if you belong to a health maintenance organization (HMO). For families who are not insured or whose coverage is not adequate, there are a number of other options worth investigating. These programs vary from locality to locality, and frequently the application processes are lengthy and frustrating. Some options worth inquiring about include: State Crippled Children's Services (in some states under the Medical Assistance program), Supplemental Security Income (SSI), administered by the Social Security Administration, Hill-Burton funding in some hospitals built with federal funds, and philanthropic organizations like the Lions and Shriners. Social workers or hospital social-service departments can be extremely helpful in these matters.

In many ways, the babyhood of an infant with spina bifida is much like that of other children. Although there obviously will be extra trips to the doctor and disappointments, such as cutting hair and shaving off new curls for a shunt revision, most things do go smoothly. Children with spina bifida need to be hugged and loved just like other little kids. They enjoy tickling games, going to grandma's, and rides in the car. Like all children they'll learn to smile, play "Pat-a-cake," recognize grandpa, and jabber and talk. Some children may proceed a little more slowly than their nonhandicapped friends, but the progression is the same. If developmental lag is a problem, an infant stimulation program and its staff can provide help to encourage language development and the maturation of other skills.

As babies grow into toddlers and preschoolers, they become more a part of the world. They get around more and find more things to talk about. The natural exuberance of this age is also found in the child with spina bifida. This is a time when it is important that mobility impairments do not interfere with opportunities to make friends and explore. A hand-pedaled bike, nursery school, or "sleep-overs" with other kids can be as important as therapy and medical intervention.

Self-confidence and a reasonable self-image are important to all children, but they are even more so for those with disabilities. These early years are the time to encourage a child to feel "OK" to be different. The resource list in the appendix includes several children's books about kids with spina bifida and other physical handicaps. They make good bedtime stories. This is not an age at which to limit children's dreams, even those that are most unrealistic. True, most kids with spina bifida won't grow up to be fire fighters, olympic athletes, or ballet dancers. But, then, neither will most other children with those fantasies. Even young children can begin to learn proper names for body parts, answers to questions about braces and walkers, and simple explanations of spina bifida.

The School-Aged Child

For children who have been in infant-stimulation or early-education programs for several years, kindergarten may not come as much of a disruption. For others it may be their first time away from the security of parents. There are two sets of tasks to be mastered by the school-aged child, academic and social. Children are responsible for mastering material covered in the curriculum, as well as getting along in a new setting with their peers. Both of these areas can be complicated for the child with spina bifida.

All children with spina bifida are entitled to an appropriate public education. Federal Law (PL94-l42) requires a school district to provide this in the least restrictive environment. Most kids with spina bifida can be "mainstreamed"—they can attend regular public-school classes. If extra help is needed, such as a bus that accommodates a wheelchair, help with intermittent catheterization, or a ramp to get safely up the front steps, the school district is obligated to provide the necessary support or at least an acceptable alternative. A school board cannot escape this responsibility, especially with the claim that modifications are too expensive or that it's only for one or two children. There are resources listed in the appendix to assist concerned parents in dealing with these matters. At times, in the past, some school districts have been uncooperative and, on occasion, parents have had to resort to court action to ensure that their child gets what he or she is entitled to.

One mechanism that helps to provide the best education for a child is the legal requirement that the school, together with the parents, write an IEP (Individual Education Plan). The IEP is a list of goals for the child to attain and the teaching methods that will be used to enable the child to do so. Ideally, the IEP is custom-made for the child. This individualized approach is especially important for the child with spina bifida, who may be vulnerable to developmental and learning problems.

Throughout this book we've stressed how striking the differences are among children with spina bifida. These variations also apply to educational expectations. Mental skills and educational development can range widely from above normal to severely retarded. There is some connection between the degree of the initial hydrocephalus, and how well it is controlled through infancy, and the child's ultimate educational abilities. Since many factors influence educational capabilities, this connection is very inexact. Among children with severe untreated hydrocephalus there is a high incidence of retardation; optimally treated hydrocephalic children appear to have fewer educational problems. However, even when the hydrocephalus is well-treated, learning problems are more common in children with spina bifida than in their classmates. Children with spina bifida seem to be much more prone to develop specific learning disabilities than other children. One area, such as reading ability, may be especially affected. For example, a child may confuse letters, mistaking "ab" for "ad." Fortunately, special help and special teaching methods are available to compensate for many of these problems. Finally, it should be emphasized that it is not reasonable to look at the mental development of present-day adults with spina bifida and past hydrocephalus as a predictor for today's children. In recent years, the outcomes of a total treatment program are much different, owing to new developments in treatment, aggressive medical therapy, special education, and support programs.

Often parents of a child with spina bifida are surprised to find their child is not doing as well at school as they had expected. Their child in early years may have seemed so "bright," very talkative and verbally skilled. A child with spina bifida may well be able to converse better than he or she can understand—the phenomenon known as "cocktail-party speech." As a consequence, there may be a significant difference between the child's tested verbal IQ and his or her performance IQ. The child's chatty manner may mask learning problems for a while. It should not be allowed to substitute for real learning.

If a child misses school owing to hospitalization, it is important that he or she keep up with classroom assignments and with his or her peer group. If the situation permits, work can be brought along, some hospitals have teachers, home-bound teaching can be arranged, and many children can return to school quickly in spite of casts or a new brace.

It is virtually impossible to predict what types of problems, if any, an individual child will have in school. Some children with spina bifida will sail along without a hitch, but the majority will be average students and may likely require some tutoring or assistance. Unfortunately, some others will be able to master little more than survival skills. No matter what a child's educational potential, it is imperative that the parents and school work together to maximize educational achievement. When the school is a reluctant participant on the team, parents' groups such as the Spina Bifida Association, the Association for Children with Learning Disabilities, and the Association for Retarded Citizens can provide assistance.

From the perspective of many childen, classes are not the most important part of the school day. They attend school primarily for the socializing. This can also be true for children with spina bifida. Ideally, they will be in a mainstreamed classroom, getting ready to live in a mainstreamed world with both disabled and able-bodied friends. This is the time to increase a child's knowledge of spina bifida and his or her ability to explain it to others. Spina bifida may be a good topic for show-and-tell or a book report. At the same time that a child with spina bifida is building friendships in school, establishment of outside interests and activities is also important. The child should have a chance to get to meet successful disabled adults, who can serve as role models. One fun way to do this is through the wheelchair athletic leagues which exist in many areas. There are also wheelchair junior leagues in such sports as basketball, track and field, and floor hockey.

One surprising transition that a child may make as he or she gets older is from crutch-walking to a wheelchair. Often children ask to make the switch when they feel the positives of a chair (speed and distance) outweigh the negatives (inaccessible areas and being different). A child's increasing size, without a parallel increase in muscle strength, may mean that for the older child, more work is required to go the same distance. Greater utilization of a wheelchair should not be regarded as a defeat. Parents can ease tensions by avoiding phrases such as "confined to a wheelchair." There are many lightweight "racy" wheelchairs on the market that have a lot to offer independent older children.

Another area that is important to all children, and especially to those with spina bifida, is the development of a sense of responsibility. When their handicapped child is a toddler or small child, it's often easier for parents to do something (or everything) for him or her. However, if the child is deprived of the opportunity to do even simple tasks, such as picking up toys or making a bed, he or she doesn't get a chance to become a contributing member of the family. When a child has a disability, there often exist lesser expectations, first on the parents' part and then on the child's. In this unhealthy situation, "pitching in" around the house never becomes an issue. Without some kind of expectations, it is hard for a child to develop a sense of responsibility. One helpful guideline is to expect a child with spina bifida to do the same tasks required of brothers and sisters at the same age. With this sort of philosophy, occasional adaptations need to be made. For example, although it may be cumbersome to assign daily dog-walking chores to a child with spina bifida, feeding and grooming Fido may be reasonable alternatives. With maturity it is extremely important that the child with spina bifida learns personal care, such as self-catheterization and brace checks. As the child nears adolescence, involvement in and understanding of plans for medical care is reasonable and beneficial.

As a child with spina bifida gets older and as the limitations and the degree of impaired mobility become more apparent, it may be necessary to make some changes in the house, chiefly to make it more accessible. A young child may be able to safely crawl up a flight of stairs to the bedrooms, but a young teen may find this too tedious and understandably undignified. In a situation such as this, some families shift the child's bedroom to the ground floor or install a stair lift, while others choose to move to a single-story home. If a child needs to use a wheelchair inside the house, the child's growth may necessitate the use of a larger chair and, as a consequence, widening of doorways. The bathroom is often one of the least accessible and least safe areas in the home. The resources listed in the appendix include information on remodeling and design specifications that will make a home more convenient and accessible for the disabled person.

The Adolescent and Adult

The teen years are a period of turmoil for most children and their families; spina bifida provides no protection from this upheaval. Once again, it is important to remember the vast differences from one individual to the next. The course of this trying period of time is influenced greatly by many of the patterns that have been previously established during childhood. A child who has been expected to take responsibility for household chores and personal hygiene is in a different position from one who has been "babied" for years.

Personal hygiene can provide a lot of parent-child conflict during the teen years. While an able-bodied boy may irritate his father because he doesn't change his socks or wash his hair, this will have little effect on the boy's health. However, if a teenager with spina bifida decides not to check beneath his or her braces for reddened areas or not to change soiled underwear for a week, there is a risk of pressure sores and the complications that accompany them.

Self-esteem is another difficult issue during adolescence. Teens want to fit in. Their appearance is very important, and they are eager to be accepted by their peers. Interest in members of the opposite sex develops. In this regard, young people with spina bifida are no different from others. Moreover, they have tangible negatives in their life on which to blame problems. Parents need to remember the trauma of their own adolescence and recall that even without a disability, times can be tough. It's important not to fall into the trap of pitying a young person with a disability. The activities in which the school-aged child joined and participated during earlier years now become even more important. Because the teenager with spina bifida has limited mobility, chauffeuring demands on parents increase and, in many cases, actually become burdensome.

Many young people with spina bifida can learn to drive, provided their sense of responsibility and intellectual development are adequate. Often the car must be modified—for example, hand controls may be needed. Information on these adaptations, as well as on driver-education classes, is often available through the state Department of Vocational Rehabilitation (DVR) and adult rehabilitation facilities. If a school system offers driver-training courses to other students, it may also be obligated to teach those with disabilities. It pays to ask before the student reaches the appropriate age, to enable the system to prepare or adapt. In addition, many metropolitan areas have bus transportation services for individuals with disabilities. Often a young person with spina bifida can master these systems and become reasonably mobile and independent.

Young people with spina bifida experience the changes of puberty such as menstruation, breast development, voice changes, and beard growth just as other teenagers do. Although there is often concern that these changes occur "too early" or "too late," the range of normal for the general population is so broad that most individuals fall well within the limits. Most likely menstruation will not have to be dealt with any differently in a young woman with spina bifida than it is with young women without disabilities.

Young people with spina bifida have the biological drives that will make them want to love and be loved, touch and be touched, and care for others and be cared for in return. From earliest childhood, children enjoy being patted, hugged, and cuddled by members of their family. As they get older, they begin to return these gestures, and as they mature, they want to share them with others. Sexuality is the desire for contact and relationship. It includes sexual behavior such as intercourse, but it is not limited to the sexual act. Often discussions of sexuality are limited to concerns about sexual anatomy and reproduction. When talking to people with spina bifida, it is important not to limit the discussions to "plumbing."

In our culture, it is often assumed that sexuality will not be part of the life of a person with a disability, and so some parents choose to avoid this area with their handicapped children in order to "spare their feelings." Although parents and other relatives will often tease children with phrases such as

"I'll dance at your wedding" or "I hope your children are as naughty as you are," kids with physical problems often don't get these and similar messages. They grow up assuming there will be a void in their lives that other people fill with friends, lovers, spouses, and children. Often disabled children grow up without sex education. The topic may be covered in a physical-education class from which they've been excused, or at a slumber party to which they didn't get invited. Or there may be no discussion at all. This combination of lack of encouragement and lack of education can make those with a disability very vulnerable both to sadness and to exploitation.

There is relatively little information available on sexuality which is specific to individuals with spina bifida. Until recent times, few individuals with neural tube defects survived to adulthood and those who did lived very sheltered lives. However, there is information that can be applied which actually relates to spinal-cord injury. Sexuality is one more area in which function is partly determined by the amount of damage sustained by the feeling (touch and pain) and motor (muscle/moving) nerves. Since the nerves to the genital areas are low on the spinal cord, much the same as the bladder, sensation in the genital areas is very frequently affected when a person has spina bifida (Figure 3). However, since sexual responsiveness has visual and psychological-emotional dimensions, and since it also involves stimulation of body parts other than the genitals, simply commenting on the nerves that reach the genitalia does not adequately deal with the situation.

In fact, women with spina bifida can have satisfying sex lives. They can be loving partners, have sexual intercourse, experience orgasm, become pregnant, and carry a pregnancy to term. The higher the initial lesion, the less likely a woman is to be able to feel sensations in the area around the vagina and in the genital area. Men with spina bifida can also have rich sex lives. They can be loving partners, have sexual intercourse, and experience orgasm. In men, the higher the initial lesion, the less likely a man is to achieve an erection of the penis from touch, to ejaculate, and to impregnate a woman. But again, experience with patients who have suffered a spinal injury has shown that there are many ways to compensate.

It is important to remember that there is immense variation among people regarding sexuality. Also, this is an area in which the individual's attitudes and self-esteem have at least as much of an impact as does physical ability. (The resource listing in the appendix includes information on sexuality.)

One of the major tasks of everyone's adolescence and young adulthood is to become an independent person. There are struggles and pain on both the child's and the parents' parts, but there is also joy. For an individual with spina bifida, the struggle may be more difficult. A young person may have depended on parents for help with personal care that others may have managed alone for years. A mother may still have the same need to protect "her baby" as she did when first hearing of the child's birth defect. A father may see how naive his child is compared to others of the same age and will fear the hurt that the world can inflict. Still, there is a lot of joy on both sides in living independently, "just like everybody else." The preparation for independent living should begin when a child is young. Developing self-esteem and responsibility cannot be stressed too strongly. Many regions now have programs of transitional living to help a young person with a disability to achieve basic living skills and attitudes that were missed along the way. Now, more than ever, there is accessible housing, and for those who still need a little extra help, personal care attendants can be hired. Planning for adulthood should proceed for a young person with spina bifida just as for any adult. There is no reason to assume that a healthy individual with a myelomeningocele won't live into old age.

Most individuals with spina bifida are capable of holding a job. Employment will provide health insurance, and it is essential that an adult with spina bifida always has adequate health insurance, through an employee benefit program, a private policy, or a government program. For the individual with spina bifida, employment often has some very practical limitations. People with neural tube defects do not have promising careers ahead of them as professional athletes, or as air force pilots. But there is a wide variety of interesting and challenging occupational skills they can acquire. Once again, lack of motivation and expectation can have as great an impact as an individual's physical limitations. The Department of Vocational Rehabilitation is often of assistance and is a good resource when considering later employment and career opportunities.

Spina bifida, and the problems associated with it, can have an enormous impact on the individual and his or her family. However, with an aggressive treatment program involving multidisciplinary care, the problems can be minimized and the child's potential—physical, emotional, and intellectual— can be maximized. This can happen only with the support of the child's family, most especially the parents. They are best prepared to provide the care that is required and to make the decisions that must be made. We hope that this book has provided some assistance to those who have these responsibilities.

Appendix

USEFUL TERMS TO KNOW

Alpha-Feto Protein: A special protein (chemical) in the fetus's circulation. When there is an open neural tube defect, this protein leaks into the amniotic fluid surrounding the baby and then into the mother's blood.

Amniocentesis: Removing a sample of amniotic fluid from around the baby, usually for diagnostic purposes such as measuring alpha-feto protein or other chemicals or cells.

Anencephaly: A fatal neural tube defect in which the brain is undeveloped or severely malformed.

Arnold-Chiari Malformation: A maldevelopment of the brain at the base of the skull near its junction with the spinal cord. Often associated with hydrocephalus and spina bifida.

Artificial Sphincter: A device implanted surgically in the body to make bladder and urination control possible.

Bladder: A hollow, muscular, walled organ in the pelvis that holds and stores urine.

Catheter: A tube used to drain fluid from a body cavity, e.g., the bladder or a brain ventricle.

CT (Computed Tomography) Scan: Also called CAT scan or Computerized Axial Tomography. A procedure in which x-rays and a computer are used to produce cross-sectional views of the body part being studied. Often employed in viewing the head or brain to check for hydrocephalus.

Contracture: A scarred, permanent muscle contraction which leaves a joint fixed and immobile. Usually results when one muscle group is functional while its opposing group is paralyzed.

Crede: An external downward abdominal pressure used to assist in emptying the bladder.

CSF: See Spinal Fluid.

Decubitus Ulcer: See Pressure Sore.

Electroencephalogram (EEG): A recording of the patterns and rhythmic electrical activity of the brain. Often done to understand more about seizures, their location and origin in the brain.

Epilepsy: An ongoing occurrence of seizures requiring medication for control.

Esotropia: Crossed eyes.

Fontanel: The soft spot on an infant's skull where the individual bones of the skull are separated.

Hydrocephalus: A condition in which the volume and pressure of the spinal fluid in the brain cavities' ventricles are increased owing to blockage of fluid circulation or absorption.

IEP (Individual Education Plan): A plan specifying educational goals and the means for reaching them, as required by law for every child in a special-education program.

Intermittent Catheterization: Insertion of a narrow soft tube (catheter) into the bladder for emptying on a regular schedule.

IVP (Intravenous Pyelogram): A special x-ray dye study used as one means of assessing kidney function.

Kidney: An organ deep in the mid-back that removes toxic wastes and substances from the body and eliminates them in the urine.

Kyphosis: A forward curvature of the spine which may produce a hump on the back.

Mainstreaming: Placing a disabled child in an educational program or classroom within the regular classroom and school setting.

Meningocele: A sac on the back containing little or no nerve tissue. A lesser variant of meningomyelocele (myelomeningocele).

Meningomyelocele: See Myelomeningocele.

Myelodysplasia: Abnormal development of the spinal cord. Used interchangeably with myelomeningocele or the more general term spina bifida.

Myelomeningocele (mie-lo-me-ning-go-seal): An abnormal development of the spinal cord, in which the spinal cord and nerves are open or contained in a thin-walled sac on the lower back, commonly used interchangeably with meningomyelocele or with the general term spina bifida.

Nerves: See Spinal Nerves.

Nervous System: The brain, spinal cord, and nerves.

Neural Tube Defect (NTD): An abnormality in the structural development of the brain or spinal cord. Includes myelomeningocele, encephalocele, and anencephaly.

Neurological: Pertaining to the nerves or the nervous system (brain, spinal cord, and nerves).

Orthosis: A brace.

Pressure Sore: Also called in its severest form a decubitus ulcer. The latter is a deep wound (often infected) found in areas where an individual often has no sensation or feeling. In its most minor form, it is a small skin blister.

Range of Motion Exercises: Moving of the joints throughout their normal motions by another person.

Reflux: Fluid traveling backward in contrast to the normal direction of its flow, as when urine backs up from the bladder into the kidneys.

Scoliosis: A side-to-side curvature of the spine.

Seizure: Inappropriate electrical activity in the brain, often producing bodily jerking movements or some type of sensory phenomena. In their minor form, there may be only a momentary loss of attention or consciousness.

Shunt: A thin tube draining fluid from one space to another. In hydrocephalus, a tube that drains from the brain cavity (ventricle) to another body area.

Shunt Tap: The sterile sampling of spinal fluid (CSF) from a shunt reservoir for pressure measurement or examination and analysis.

Spina Bifida (spi-nah bif-ida): A general term for meningomyelocele or myelomeningocele. In the strictest sense, a defect or split in the formation of a vertebra.

Spina Bifida Cystica: A severe type of spina bifida, including myelomeningocele.

Spina Bifida Occulta: A common condition in which a portion of the vertebra covering the spinal canal and spinal cord is malformed, but without spinal cord involvement or cyst formation—a very minor type of spina bifida.

Spinal Column: A series of individual bones (vertebrae) in the neck and back supporting the body and head, and containing the spinal cord. Commonly referred to as the spine.

Spinal Fluid: The clear water-like fluid surrounding and contained within the brain cavities, and for its protection and support. Commonly referred to as CSF.

Spinal Nerves: Nerves arising regularly at each level of the spinal column and passing to a specific body area or part for muscle movement or contraction (motor nerves), as well as from the same areas, to receive sensation such as touch, pain, or temperature (sensory nerves).

Subluxation: Dislocation of a joint.

Ultrasound: A special test using high-frequency sound waves to ''see'' inside the body or head.

Ureter: The conduit (or tube) within the body draining urine from the kidneys to the bladder.

Urethra: The conduit (or tube) draining urine from the bladder to outside the body.

Urinary Diversion: An operation in which a small piece of intestine is used to create a conduit for urinary drainage to the abdominal wall.

Vertebra: A single supporting bone of the spine.

Vertebrae: All the supporting bones of the spine.

Vesicostomy: A surgical opening of the bladder onto the abdominal wall.

WHO'S WHO IN SPINA BIFIDA CARE PROGRAMS

Many professionals may become involved in the care of a child with spina bifida.

Genetic Counselor: A health professional who provides information about hereditary conditions.

Geneticist: A health professional who specializes in hereditary conditions.

Intern: A physician in his/her first year following medical school, currently referred to as a first-year resident.

Neonatologist: A special type of pediatrician who has particular expertise in the care of the newborn.

Neurologist: A physician who specializes in the diagnosis of problems of the nervous system and the treatment of medical (nonsurgical) diseases of the brain, spinal cord, and nerves.

Neurosurgeon: A surgeon who specializes in surgery of the nervous system (brain, spinal cord, and nerves).

Nurse Clinician: A registered nurse (RN) with a special interest and expertise in a particular area of medical care.

Occupational Therapist: A member of the health-care team who evaluates and suggests methods for dealing with the impact of disabilities on arms and hands.

Ophthalmologist: A physician who specializes in medical and surgical conditions of the eye. Commonly referred to as an ''eye doctor'' and not to be confused with an optometrist, who prescribes corrective glasses, or an optician, who makes and fits glasses.

Orthopedic Surgeon (Orthopedist): A physician who specializes in the problems and surgery of bones and joints. Commonly referred to as a ''bone doctor.''

Orthotist: An individual who works with the health-care team and who makes and fits braces.

Pediatric Endocrinologist: A pediatrician who specializes in growth disorders and hormone or glandular diseases of children.

Pediatrician: A physician who specializes in the care of infants and children. Commonly referred to as a ''baby doctor.''

Physiatrist: A physician who specializes in treating disabilities and in rehabilitation.

Physical Therapist: A member of the health-care team who provides treatment and instruction to build strength and range of motion in order to encourage mobility.

Plastic Surgeon: A physician who specializes in the surgical repair and reconstruction of deformed tissues.

Primary Care Physician: A physician (often a family practitioner or pediatrician) who provides the majority of initial health care and who coordinates treatment by specialists.

Public Health Nurse: A registered nurse who provides nursing and health care education and evaluation at home.

Radiologist: A physician who specializes in the interpretation and use of x-rays for diagnostic tests.

Resident: A physician who is in an educational program to become a specialist.

Social Worker: An individual who provides counseling about emotional, social, and financial problems. In the hospital setting, a member of the health-care team.

Special Education Teacher: A specially trained teacher who educates children who have handicaps which affect their ability to learn.

Speech and Language Pathologist: An individual who evaluates a person's ability to speak and to understand speech and who suggests and provides appropriate therapy.

Urologist: A physician who specializes in problems and surgery of the urinary tract.

HELPFUL ORGANIZATIONS

Many groups provide information and support to individuals dealing with handicapping conditions. The following is a list of national organizations concerned with spina bifida. Most of these societies have state and local chapters which can be found by contacting the association office through the telephone book. Many spina bifida clinics and school programs have groups that provide support and information to families.

Spina Bifida Association of America
1700 Rockville Pike
Suite 540
Rockville, Maryland 20852
312-663-1562

This group and its state and local chapters have the most relevant information on spina bifida.

March of Dimes Birth Defects Foundation
1275 Mamoroneck Avenue
White Plains, New York 10605
914-428-7100

Association for Children and Adults with Learning Disabilities
4156 Library Road
Pittsburgh, Pennsylvania 15234

Association for Retarded Citizens
2501 Avenue J
Arlington, Texas 76011

National Easter Seal Society
2023 West Ogden Avenue
Chicago, Illinois 60612

National Wheelchair Athletic Association
40-24 62nd Street
Woodside, New York 11377

Parents' Campaign for Handicapped Children
  and Youth/Closer Look
1201 16th Street N.W.
Washington, D.C. 20036

Canada

The Hugh MacMillan Center
350 Rumsey Road
Toronto, Ontario M4D 1R8
416-425-6220

The Spina Bifida Associaion of Canada
633 Wellington Crescent
Winnipeg, Manitoba R3M 0A8
204-452-7580

Spina Bifida and Hydrocephalus
  Association of Ontario
55 Queen Street East
Toronto, Ontario M5C 1R5
416-364-1871

Spinal Cord Society of Canada
P.O. Box 707
King City, Ontario L06 1K0
416-833-0984

USEFUL BOOKS

Everybody needs help to get through life. When a child has spina bifida, the family needs an extra boost. These extra hands can be found among relatives, in the hospital, in infant programs, at church, in support groups, and even at the public library. Lists of resources can never be complete, since new ones are always emerging. But the following books should provide a good place to start.

About Spina Bifida and Other Physical Disabilities

Anderson, E. and Spain, B. *The Child with Spina Bifida*. Love Publishing Company, Denver, Colorado, 1977.

Clopton, N. *Caring for Your Child with Spina Bifida*. Eterna Press, Oak Brook, Illinois, 1981.

Forrai, M. and Russel, M. *A Look at Physical Handicaps*. Lerner Publications Company, Minneapolis, Minnesota, 1976.

Henderson, M. and Dynhotdy, F. *Care of the Infant with Myelomeningocele and Hydrocephalus*. University of Iowa, Iowa City, Iowa, 1975.

Myers, G., Cerone S., and A. Olson, eds. *A Guide for Helping the Child with Spina Bifida*. Charles C Thomas Publisher, Springfield, Illinois, 1981.

Nakos, E. and Taylor, S. *Early Development of the Child with Myelomeningocele: A Parent's Guide*. Children's Hospital Medical Center, Cincinnati, Ohio, 1977. Free!

Reid, R. *My Children, My Children*. Harcourt Brace Jovanovich, New York, 1977.

Swinyard, C. *The Child with Spina Bifida*. Spina Bifida Association of America, Chicago, Illinois, 1977.

About Coping When the Going Gets Tough

Dougan, T., Isbell, L., and Vyas, P. *We Have Been There*. Abingdon Press, Nashville, Tennessee, 1982. By parents of mentally retarded children.

Kushner, H. *When Bad Things Happen to Good People*. Schocken Books, New York, 1981. By a rabbi whose son died after a long illness.

Mitchell, J. *Taking on the World*. Harcourt Brace Jovanovich, New York, 1982. Subtitled *Empowering Strategies for Parents of Children with Disabilities*.

Murphy, A. *Special Children, Special Parents*. Prentice-Hall, Inc., Englewood-Cliffs, New Jersey, 1981. Subtitled *Personal Issues with Handicapped Children*.

Powell, T. and Ogle, P. A. *Brothers and Sisters—A Special Part of Exceptional Families*. Paul H. Brookes Publishing Co., Baltimore, Maryland, 1985.

Russell, P. *The Wheelchair Child, How Handicapped Children Can Enjoy Life to Its Fullest*. Prentice-Hall, Inc., Englewood-Cliffs, New Jersey, 1983.

Practical Suggestions

Barish, F. *Frommer's A Guide for the Disabled Traveler*. Simon and Schuster, Inc., New York, 1984.

Caston, D. *Easy-to-Make Aids for Your Handicapped Child. A Guide for Parents and Teachers*. Prentice-Hall, Inc., Englewood Cliffs, New Jersey, 1981.

Gary, J. *How to Create Interiors for the Disabled: A Guide for Family and Friends*. Pantheon Books, New York, 1978.

Hotte, E. *Self-Help Clothing for Children Who have Physical Disabilities*. The National Easter Seal Society for Crippled Children and Adults, Chicago, Illinois, 1979.

McConkey, R. and Jeffree, D. *Making Toys for Handicapped Children, A Guide for Parents and Teachers*. Prentice-Hall, Inc., Englewood Cliffs, New Jersey, 1981.

Moore, C., Morton, K., and Southard, A. *A Reader's Guide for Parents of Children with Mental, Physical or Emotional Disabilities*. The

Maryland State Planning Council on Developmental Disabilities, Baltimore, Maryland, 1983. An extensive annotated bibliography.

Te Grootenhuis, G. and Jorstad, C. *Street Wheeling Manual*, Metropolitan Center for Independent Living, St. Paul, Minnesota, 1982. All about electric wheelchairs.

For Children

Babe, B. *The Balancing Girl*. E. P. Dutton, New York, 1981.

Bennet, C. *Giant Steps for Steven*. After School Exchange, Mayfield Heights, Ohio, 1980.

Biklen, D. and Sokoloff, M. *What Do You Do When Your Wheelchair Gets a Flat Tire?* Scholastic's Feeling Fine, Englewood Cliffs, New Jersey, 1978.

Fanshawe, E. *Rachel*. Bradbury Press, Scarsdale, New York, 1977.

Fassler, J. *Howie Helps Himself*. Albert Whitman and Company, Chicago, Illinois, 1975.

Frevert, P. *It's Okay to Look at Jamie*. Creative Education, Inc., Mankato, Minnesota, 1983.

Howe, J. and Warshaw, M. *The Hospital Book*. Crown Publishers, Inc., New York, 1981.

Lasker, J. *Nick Joins In*. Albert Whitman and Company, Chicago, Illinois, 1980.

Mitchell, J. *See Me More Clearly*. Harcourt Brace Jovanovich, New York, 1980.

Nadas, B. *Danny's Song*. Hubbard, Northbrook, Illinois, 1975. From the Mister Rogers people.

Savitz, H. *Run, Don't Walk*. Accent Special Publications, Bloomington, Illinois, 1979. For teens.

Stein, S. *About Handicaps: An Open Family Book for Parents and Children Together*. Walker and Company, New York, 1974.

White, P. *Janet at School*. Harper and Row, New York, 1978.

School

Anderson, W., Chitwood, S., and Hayden, D., eds. *Negotiating the Special Education Maze, A Guide for Parents and Teachers*. Prentice-Hall, Inc., Englewood Cliffs, New Jersey, 1981.

Cutler, B. *Unraveling the Special Education Maze*. Research Press, Champaign, Illinois, 1981.

Sunderlin, S., ed. *The Most Enabling Environment Education Is for All Children*. Association for Childhood Education International, Washington, D.C., 1979.

Sexuality

Ayrault, E. *Sex, Love and the Physically Handicapped*. Continuum Publishing Company, New York, 1981.

Blum, G. and Blum, B. *Feeling Good About Yourself*. Academic Therapy Publications, Novato, California, 1977.

Cornelius, D. et al. *Who Cares? A Handbook on Sex Education and Counseling Services for Disabled People*. University Park Press, Baltimore, Maryland, 1982.

Duffy, Y. *All Things Are Possible*. A. J. Garvin and Associates, Ann Arbor, Michigan, 1981.

Images of Ourselves: Women with Disabilities Talking. Routledge and Kegan Paul, Boston, 1981.

McKee L. and Blacklidge, V. *An Easy Guide for Parents*. Research Press, Champaign, Illinois, 1981. Subtitled *A Book for Parents of People with Mental Handicaps*.

INDEX

INDEX

Adoption, placement of newborns for, 9

Alpha Feto Protein (AFP): defined, 73; testing for presence of in amniotic fluid, 18-19

Amniocentesis: defined, 73; and testing for Alpha Feto Protein (AFP), 18-19

Anencephaly: defined, 20, 73; incidence of, 20

Ankle-foot orthoses (AFO): as aid to walking, 42; braces for treating club foot, 36

Arnold-Chiari Malformation, defined, 73

Australia, survey of lumbar defects in, 14

Bladder control: defined, 73; influence of sensory nerves on, 13; in newborn, 8

Bladder problems: caused by nerve damage, 44-48; Crede maneuver, 45-46; and kidney infections, 45; reflux, 45

Blood urea nitrogen (BUN), testing for levels of, 46

Bowel control: influence of sensory and motor nerves on, 13; in newborn, 8; problems with, 48-49

Brain: anatomy of normal, 23-24; part of central nervous system, 3; and use of nerves, 11

Catheter, defined, 73

Catheterization, intermittent: defined, 74; as treatment for urinary incontinence, 47, 48

Central nervous system: composition of, 3; controlled by genes, 16; defined, 3, 75

Cerebrospinal fluid (CSF): in brain, 23; defined, 76; obstruction of, 24; stopping leakage of with surgery, 9

Children and Adults with Learning Disabilities, Association for, 63-64, 81

Choroid plexus, defined, 24

Club foot (*Talipes equinovarus*): braces, as treatment for, 36-37; casting, as treatment for, 35-36; defined, 35; surgery, as treatment for, 37

Computerized tomography (CT): defined, 73; test for hydrocephalus, 8, 25-27

cystica, 4; damage to, 7; as part of central nervous system, 3
Spinal deformities, 42; kyphosis, 43; scoliosis, 43
Spinal fluid. *See* Cerebrospinal fluid
Spinal nerves, defined, 11, 76
Subluxation: defined, 37, 76; treatment for, 38

Talipes equinovarus. See Club foot
Toilet training, 47

Ultrasound: defined, 76; test for determining hydrocephalus, 8, 27; test for urinary tract, 46
Ureter, defined, 76
Urethra, defined, 76

Urinary diversion, defined, 76
Urinary infection, testing for with catheter, 46
Urological system, function of, 44
Urologist: defined, 44; importance of consulting, 46

Ventricles: expanding in hydrocephalus, 25-27; as part of brain, 23-24
Vertebra(ae), defined, 76
Vesicostomy, defined, 77
Vision problems, 55-56
Vocational Rehabilitation, Department of (DVR), 67, 70
Voiding cystourethrogram (VCUG), test for bladder, 47

BETH-ANN BLOOM is a genetic counselor at St. Paul Ramsey Medical Center and Gillette Children's Hospital in St. Paul, Minnesota. She received her M.S. from Sarah Lawrence College, New York.

EDWARD L. SELJESKOG is a professor of neurosurgery at the University of Minnesota Medical School. He has contributed chapters to numerous medical books and publishes regularly in neurosurgical journals.

DATE DUE